# Stem Cells

# Stem Cells

**Eapen Cherian** MDS
Reader
Department of Oral Pathology
and Forensic Odontology
Pushpagiri College of Dental Sciences
Thiruvalla, Kerala, India

*Co-authors*

**G Nandhini** MDS
Senior Lecturer
Department of Oral and
Maxillofacial Pathology
SRM Dental College
Chennai, Tamil Nadu, India

**Anil Kurian** BDS PGDCR
Researcher
Department of Oral Pathology
and Forensic Odontology
Pushpagiri College of Dental Sciences
Thiruvalla, Kerala, India

*Foreword*

**K Rajkumar**

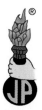

**JAYPEE BROTHERS MEDICAL PUBLISHERS (P) LTD**

New Delhi • Panama City • London

*Published by*

**Jaypee Brothers Medical Publishers (P) Ltd**

*Corporate Office*

4838/24, Ansari Road, Daryaganj, **New Delhi** 110 002, India
Phone: +91-11-43574357, Fax: +91-11-43574314
Website: www.jaypeebrothers.com

*Offices in India*

- **Ahmedabad**, e-mail: ahmedabad@jaypeebrothers.com
- **Bengaluru**, e-mail: bangalore@jaypeebrothers.com
- **Chennai**, e-mail: chennai@jaypeebrothers.com
- **Delhi**, e-mail: jaypee@jaypeebrothers.com
- **Hyderabad**, e-mail: hyderabad@jaypeebrothers.com
- **Kochi**, e-mail: kochi@jaypeebrothers.com
- **Kolkata**, e-mail: kolkata@jaypeebrothers.com
- **Lucknow**, e-mail: lucknow@jaypeebrothers.com
- **Mumbai**, e-mail: mumbai@jaypeebrothers.com
- **Nagpur**, e-mail: nagpur@jaypeebrothers.com

*Overseas Offices*

- **Central America Office, Panama City, Panama**, Ph: 001-507-317-0160
  e-mail: cservice@jphmedical.com, Website: www.jphmedical.com
- **Europe Office, UK**, Ph: +44 (0) 2031708910
  e-mail: info@jpmedpub.com

*Stem Cells*

© 2011, Jaypee Brothers Medical Publishers

*First Edition :* **2011**
ISBN  978-93-5025-060-0
Typeset at JPBMP typesetting unit
Printed in India

*Dedicated to*
**My Dear Family**

# Foreword

It is a privilege to write a foreword for the book titled *Stem Cells* authored by Dr Eapen Cherian, Reader, Department of Oral Pathology and Forensic Odontology, Pushpagiri College of Dental Sciences, Thiruvalla, Kerala, India and co-authored by Dr G Nandhini, Senior Lecturer, Department of Oral and Maxillofacial Pathology, SRM Dental College, Chennai, Tamil Nadu, India and Dr Anil Kurian, Researcher, Department of Oral Pathology and Forensic Odontology, Pushpagiri College of Dental Sciences, Thiruvalla, Kerala, India.

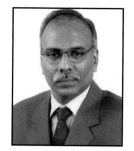

Stem cells are such a fascinating field in science with tremendous scope to dramatically change the treatment of human diseases. Every organ and tissue is made up of specialized cells that originate from a pool of stem cells. Stem cells play a vital role in regenerating organs and tissues that are injured or lost every day, such as our skin, hair, blood and the lining of our gut. Knowledge about stem cells is central to understanding not just normal development, but also human disease and injury, and for using this knowledge to develop new therapies.

This textbook provides a comprehensive and complete review of what you need to know about stem cells. This book will not only serve as a source of information to the scientific fraternity, but also to the general public. The authors have made every attempt to make it an excellent compilation.

I wish them all success in their endeavors.

**K Rajkumar** BSc MDS
Professor and Head
Department of Oral and Maxillofacial Pathology and Microbiology
Editor-in-Chief, STREAMDENT—SRM University Journal of Dental Sciences
SRM Dental College, Ramapuram, Chennai
Tamil Nadu, India

# Preface

It is with immense pleasure and satisfaction that I present the first edition of *Stem Cells* to students, researchers and practitioners in the medical arena.

The subject *Stem Cells* has assumed the status of a specialty only recently. With the rapid growth of this evolving subject, I felt the need for a book presenting all relevant information currently available; comprehensive enough to present relevant facts to the searching mind. Currently, very few books have been written with the objective to present this subject to researchers of the medical field.

It is hoped that this book will be a useful asset to fulfil the need of medical researchers in their quest to experiment into the ever dynamic opportunity that the world of *Stem Cells* present.

**Eapen Cherian**

# Acknowledgments

I would like to acknowledge with gratitude to my co-authors Dr G Nandhini and Dr Anil Kurian for the valuable contributions they have made in successfully completing this book. I gratefully acknowledge the encouragement and advice of my beloved teacher and mentor Prof Dr K Rajkumar, Head, Department of Oral and Maxillofacial Pathology and Microbiology, SRM Dental College, Chennai, Tamil Nadu, India and also for his valuable and constant support in all my professional endeavors throughout my life. I must acknowledge Dr Oommen Aju Jacob, Principal, Pushpagiri College of Dental Sciences, Thiruvalla, Kerala, India for his help in evaluating this book and making me to realize my potential. I also thank Prof Dr Alex K Varghese, Head, Department of Oral Pathology and Microbiology, Pushpagiri College of Dental Sciences for inspiring and encouraging me during the preparation of this book.

I also record my sincere gratitude to Dr Lizamma Alex, Vice Principal, Pushpagiri Institute of Medical Sciences, for her painstaking effort in correcting this work. In this connection, I would like to thank Dr Anuja Mathews, Lecturer, Pushpagiri College of Dental Sciences and my friends Dr Ramyamalini, Senior Lecturer, SRM Dental College, Dr Sudheerkanth, Senior Lecturer, Army College of Dental Sciences, Secunderabad, Andhra Pradesh, India for their constant support.

Rev Fr Philip Payyampallil, Director, Pushpagiri Medicity and Rev Fr Mathew Mazhuvancheryil, Director, Pushpagiri Research Centre deserve special mention for encouraging the publication of this book.

I would like to thank my family for their constant support.

Above all, I thank God Almighty for making me what I am and helping me to have achieved what I have achieved.

# Contents

# Introduction

Scientist for centuries, have known that certain animals can regenerate missing parts of their bodies. Humans share this ability with animals like the starfish and the newt. Although humans cannot replace a missing leg or a finger, our bodies are constantly regenerating skin, blood and other tissues. Experiments conducted in the 1950s with bone marrow, established the existence of stem cells as powerful cells that allow us to regenerate some tissues. This led to the development of bone marrow transplantation, a therapy now widely used in medicine.

## WHAT IS A STEM CELL?

Every cell in the human body can be traced back to a fertilized egg that came into existence from the union of an egg and a sperm. The human body is made up of not just one, but over 200 different types of cells and all of these cell types comes from a pool of stem cells in the early embryo.

Stem cells are unspecialized cells that develop into specialized cells, which in turn make up the different types of tissues in the human body. During the period of early development as well as later in life, various types of stem cells give rise to specialized or differentiated cells, such as the skin, blood, muscle and nerve cells, which carry out the specific functions of the body **(Figs 1.1 and 1.2)**.

In humans, *stem cells* have been identified in the inner cell mass of the early embryo, in some tissues of the fetus, the umbilical cord, the placenta and in several adult organs. In some of the adult organs, the stem cells give rise to more than one specialized cell type within that organ (e.g.: the neural stem cells give rise to three different cell types found in the brain neurons, glial cells and astrocytes) **(Figs 1.3 to 1.5)**.

## Defining Features of a Stem Cell

1. Stem cell "*self-renews*", i.e. a stem cell undergoes cell division when it is called into action. While one daughter cell remains a stem cell, the other becomes more committed to forming a particular cell type (a "committed progenitor") by a process called "asymmetric division".

2. Stem cell forms multiple cell types, i.e. "*multipotent*".

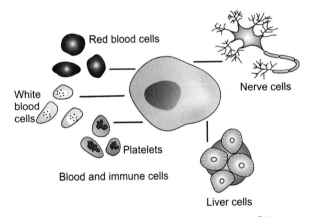

Fig. 1.1: Stem cells can differentiate into many cell types

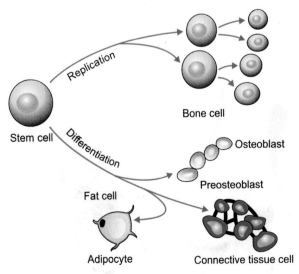

Fig. 1.2: Stem cells

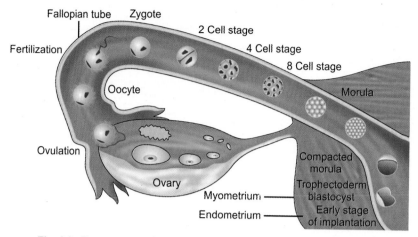

**Fig. 1.3:** From zygote to blastula—the early stages of human development

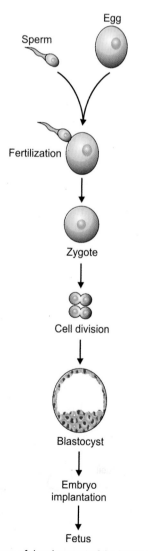

**Fig. 1.4:** Stages of development of the human embryo

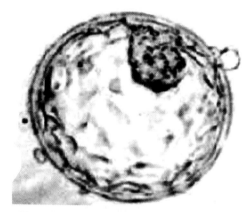

**Fig. 1.5:** A human blastocyst which is produced about 5 days fertilization

3. A single stem cell, when transplanted within the body, completely "reforms" a particular tissue.

Stem cells have thus been long regarded as undifferentiated cells capable of proliferation, self renewal, production of a large number of differentiated progeny, and regeneration of tissues **(Fig. 1.6)**.

### How do Stem Cells Look Like under the Microscope (Fig. 1.7)?

### The Ultimate in Preventative Therapies

Research shows that on comparison new stem cells are able to multiply, and make repairs, more than older stem cells, such as those existing in aging bodies. The availability of newborn stem cells, such as those we offer, makes the body maintenance processes much more active. As damaged cells are identified by the immune system, and are then

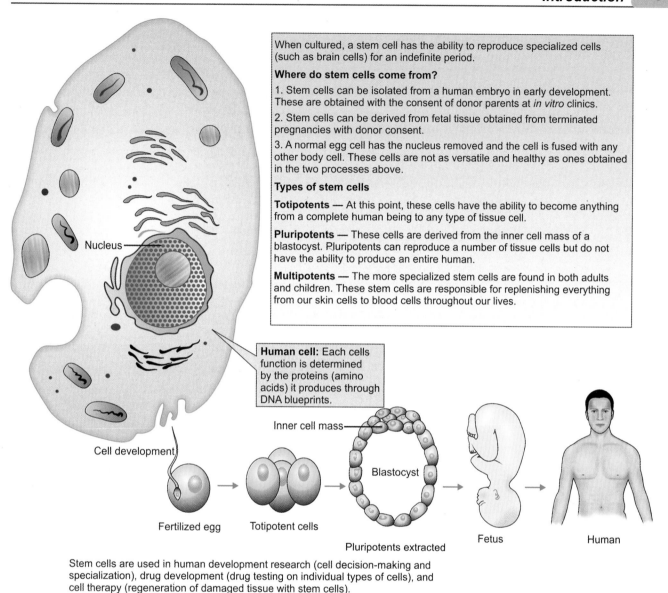

When cultured, a stem cell has the ability to reproduce specialized cells (such as brain cells) for an indefinite period.

**Where do stem cells come from?**

1. Stem cells can be isolated from a human embryo in early development. These are obtained with the consent of donor parents at *in vitro* clinics.

2. Stem cells can be derived from fetal tissue obtained from terminated pregnancies with donor consent.

3. A normal egg cell has the nucleus removed and the cell is fused with any other body cell. These cells are not as versatile and healthy as ones obtained in the two processes above.

**Types of stem cells**

**Totipotents** — At this point, these cells have the ability to become anything from a complete human being to any type of tissue cell.

**Pluripotents** — These cells are derived from the inner cell mass of a blastocyst. Pluripotents can reproduce a number of tissue cells but do not have the ability to produce an entire human.

**Multipotents** — The more specialized stem cells are found in both adults and children. These stem cells are responsible for replenishing everything from our skin cells to blood cells throughout our lives.

Nucleus

**Human cell:** Each cells function is determined by the proteins (amino acids) it produces through DNA blueprints.

Cell development

Inner cell mass

Blastocyst

Fertilized egg      Totipotent cells

Pluripotents extracted

Fetus

Human

Stem cells are used in human development research (cell decision-making and specialization), drug development (drug testing on individual types of cells), and cell therapy (regeneration of damaged tissue with stem cells).

**Fig. 1.6:** Stem cell uses

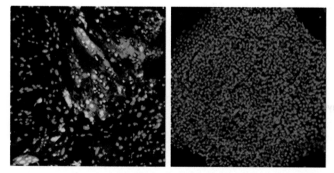

**Fig. 1.7:** Stem cell under the microscope—early human stem cells

replaced by circulating stem cells, dangerous conditions such as cancer are likely to be prevented. In fact, stem cells can be considered the ultimate preventive health measure.

Stem cell therapy involves the introduction of healthy new stem cells to, (potentially) repair, and replace damaged or lost cells. The ability to repair damaged tissues and rejuvenate aging organs makes it very effective at reversing various disease processes, as well as the signs and symptoms of aging.

# THE STEM CELL PROGRESS (FIGS 1.8 AND 1.9)

**The announcement by a US company that it has cloned a human
embryo for the first time had set off a heated debate on the ethics
of the research**

**Biotechnology company — Advanced Cell Technology Inc. based in Massachusetts,
said the research was aimed not at creating a human being but mining the
embryo for stem cells to treat diseases ranging from Parkinson's to diabetes**

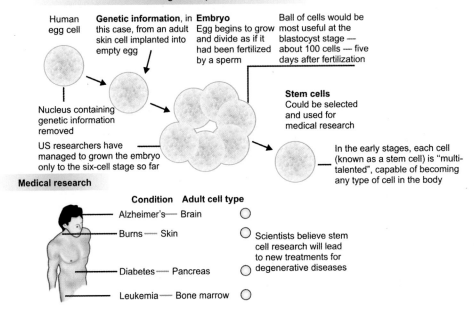

**The cloning technique**

Human egg cell

**Genetic information**, in this case, from an adult skin cell implanted into empty egg

**Embryo** Egg begins to grow and divide as if it had been fertilized by a sperm

Ball of cells would be most useful at the blastocyst stage — about 100 cells — five days after fertilization

Nucleus containing genetic information removed

US researchers have managed to grown the embryo only to the six-cell stage so far

**Stem cells** Could be selected and used for medical research

In the early stages, each cell (known as a stem cell) is "multi-talented", capable of becoming any type of cell in the body

**Medical research**

| Condition | Adult cell type |
|---|---|
| Alzheimer's | Brain |
| Burns | Skin |
| Diabetes | Pancreas |
| Leukemia | Bone marrow |

Scientists believe stem cell research will lead to new treatments for degenerative diseases

New cells implanted into patient would be identical to his or her own so would not be rejected by the body

**Fig. 1.8:** Stem cell milestone

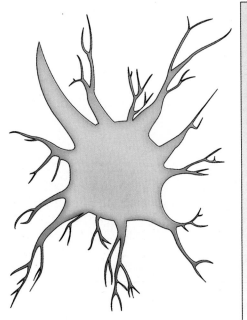

**2000**
Project ALS stem cell team transplants
a variety of stem cell types into the SOD1 mouse,
a laboratory model fo ALS.

**2001**
Project ALS funded scientists devise method
for directing the differentiation of ES (embryonic
stem) cell into functional motor neurons, the very
cells that are targeted for destruction in ALS.

**2003**
Rats paralyzed with an ALS-like syndrome regain
significant motor function after receiving an infusion of
stem cells into the spinal fluid.

**2004**
Project ALS team demonstrates that ES cell-derived
motor neurons can establish appropriate connections
with target muscles in a live animal.

**2005**
Scientists develop strategies for recruiting endogenous
stem cells—or stem cells already residing in the
body—to the ALS spinal cord.

**2006**
Project ALS opens the Jenifer Estess Laboratory for stem
cell research, the world's first privately-funded lab devoted
exclusively to the study of stem cells and ALS therapies.

**Fig. 1.9:** Virtue to stem cell

# CHAPTER 2

# *Properties and Types of Stem Cells*

## PROPERTIES OF STEM CELLS

Stem cells differ from other kinds of cells in the body. Regardless of their source, the stem cells have three general properties:

1. *Stem cells are unspecialized:* One of the fundamental properties of a stem cell is that it does not have any tissue-specific structures that allow it to perform specialized functions. A stem cell cannot:
   i. Work with its neighbors to pump blood through the body (like a heart muscle cell).
   ii. Carry molecules of oxygen through the bloodstream (like a red blood cell).
   iii. Fire electrochemical signals to other cells that allow the body to move or speak (like a nerve cell).
   Despite these, unspecialized stem cells can give rise to specialized cells including heart muscle cells, blood cells or nerve cells.
2. *Stem cells are capable of dividing and renewing themselves for long periods:* The muscle, blood or nerve cells do not replicate themselves normally. However, stem cells may replicate many times. When cells replicate themselves many times over it is called proliferation. When stem cells proliferate for many months in the laboratory, it can yield millions of cells. The cells are said to be capable of long-term self-renewal, if the resulting cells continue to be unspecialized like the parent stem cells.
3. *Stem cells can give rise to specialized cells:* When unspecialized stem cells give rise to specialized cells, the process is called differentiation. Scientists are just beginning to understand the signals inside and outside cells, which trigger stem cell differentiation. The internal signals are controlled by a cell's genes, interspersed across long strands of DNA and they carry coded instructions for every structure and function of a cell. The external signals include physical contact with neighboring cells, chemicals secreted by other cells, and certain molecules in the microenvironment **(Figs 2.1 and 2.2)**.

*Potency*: This specifies the differentiation potential of the stem cell (the potential to differentiate into different cell types) **(Figs 2.3 and 2.4)**.

*Totipotent stem cells*: Produced by the fusion of an egg and a sperm cell. The cells produced by the first few divisions of the fertilized egg are also totipotent **(Fig. 2.5)**. These cells can differentiate into both the embryonic and the extra-embryonic cell types.

*Pluripotent stem cells*: Descendants of the totipotent cells can differentiate into cells derived from any of the three germ layers **(Figs 2.6A and B)**.

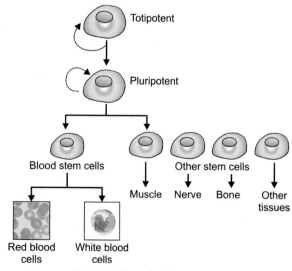

**Fig. 2.1:** Hierarchy of stem cells

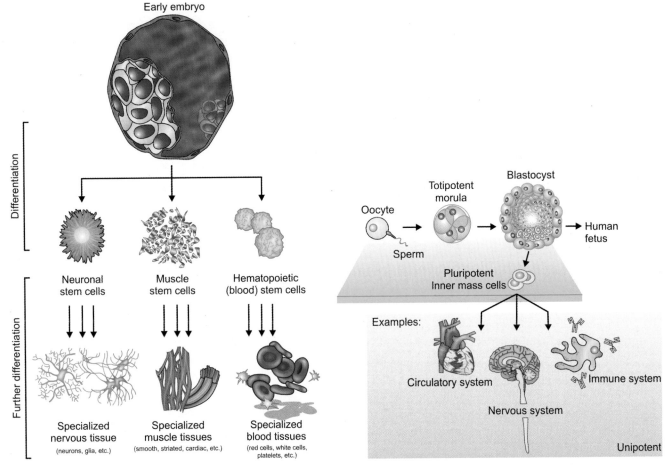

**Fig. 2.2:** Stem cell differentiation

**Fig. 2.3:** Potential of the stem cells

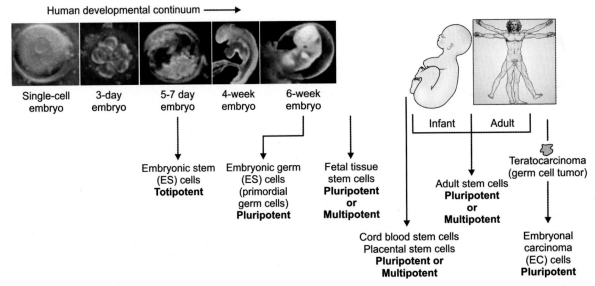

**Fig. 2.4:** Stem cells

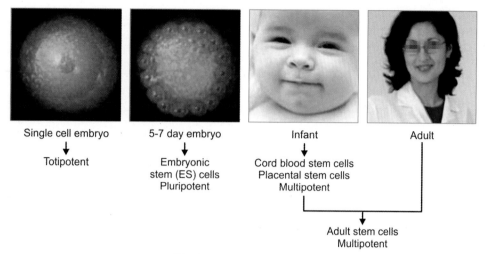

**Fig. 2.5:** Totipotent stem cells

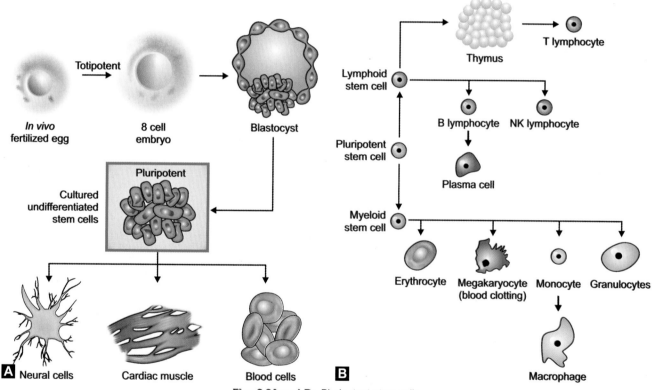

**Figs 2.6A and B:** Pluripotent stem cells

*Multipotent stem cells*: Can produce only cells of a closely related family of cells (e.g. hematopoietic stem cells differentiate into red blood cells, white blood cells, platelets, etc.) **(Fig. 2.7)**.

*Unipotent cells*: Though they can produce only one cell type, they have the property of self-renewal which distinguishes them from non-stem cells.

## TYPES OF STEM CELLS

Stem cells are found in all human beings, from the early stages of human development to the end of life. All stem cells may prove useful for medical research, but each of the different types has both promise and limitations.

1. *Embryonic stem cells*: That can be derived from a very early stage in human development, have the potential to produce all of the body's cell types **(Fig. 2.8)**.

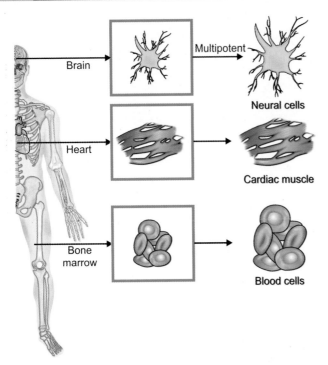

Fig. 2.7: Multipotent stem cells

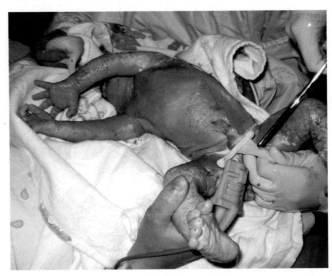

Fig. 2.9: Cord blood collection

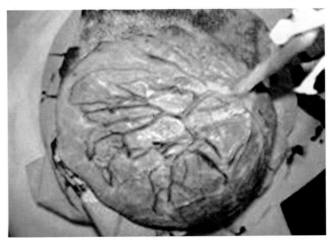

Fig. 2.10: Neonatal umbilical cord stem cells

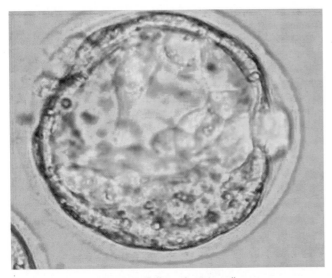

Fig. 2.8: Embryonic stem cell

2. *Adult stem cells*: That are found in certain tissues in fully developed humans, from babies to adults, may be limited to producing only certain types of specialized cells **(Fig. 2.9)**.

Recently, scientists have also identified stem cells in the umbilical cord blood and the placenta, that can give rise to various types of blood cells.

## Neonatal Umbilical Cord Stem Cells

During pregnancy, the developing fetus is fed by blood from the placenta. Blood travels through the umbilical cord and enters the baby's body at the umbilicus or navel **(Fig. 2.10)**. This blood contains large numbers of stem cells, which are actively assisting in the growth and development of the baby's body. At birth, the umbilical cord is cut, and the cord and placenta are usually discarded as medical waste. The blood remaining in the placenta and cord still contain significant numbers of stem cells, as do the placenta and cord structures themselves. To collect them, the blood is collected from the placenta and cord within five minutes of birth and placed in a special bag with a solution that prevents clotting. The blood is transported to the lab within 24 hours. Stem cells are separated from the blood using a centrifuge or other methods.

Unlike embryonic stem cells, umbilical cord stem cells are usually ignored in the media. There seems to be an organized attempt to prevent people from knowing that a readily available source of stem cells exists worldwide. This is likely because the large pharmaceutical companies seek to control the production and use of stem cells.

- These cells are *Pluripotent*, which means that they can turn into almost any cell type
- Unlike embryonic stem cells, umbilical cord stem cells do not promote tumors
- Unlike adult stem cells, umbilical cord stem cells do not cause immune reaction. Since these immature cells do not express adult tissue-type proteins (ABO, Rh, and HLA antigens) on their surfaces, these proteins do not seem to cause either an immune reaction in the recipient, or a graft vs host reaction against the recipient.
- Unlike fetal stem cells, umbilical cord stem cells do not require sacrificing a human baby or fetus.

The only accepted use for umbilical cord stem cells in establishment medicine is as a substitute for bone marrow transplant in cancer patients. After the bone marrow is destroyed by chemotherapy and radiation, cord blood stem cells have the ability to reconstitute the bone marrow. Over 5,000 cord blood cell transplants have been done for this purpose, and few, if any, side-effects have been reported.

Although the cancer specialists are only interested in re-establishing the ability to form blood, these stem cells replace much more than just bone marrow stem cells, and are likely to assist the body in recovery from cancer in other ways.

## Umbilical Cord Mesenchymal Stem Cells

The jelly-like material which fills the structure of the umbilical cord itself is rich in an additional type of stem cells, called "mesenchymal stem cells". Mesenchymal stem cells are present in cord blood but in very low concentrations **(Fig. 2.11)**. They are also present in bone marrow and help form the structure of the marrow and support the blood-forming cells there. These cells are also multipotent, and are able to differentiate into progenitor cells representing all three layers of the embryo. This means that an additional rich source of multipotent stem cells is now available.

Without further processing, mesenchymal cells readily differentiate into cells which repair bone, fat, joints, cartilage, tendons and connective tissue. With further processing, these cells have already been converted into nerve cells or brain liver and pancreas precursor cells. They have treated Parkinson's disease in rats, and have rebuilt kidney damaged tissue. Thus, it appears that these mesenchymal stem cells

are at least as exciting as the umbilical cord blood stem cells in rebuilding the many structures and organs of the body.

## Technology of Stem Cell Therapy

### Collecting the Cord Blood (Fig. 2.12)

Potential donors are prescreened for possible blood-borne infections or for risky behavior. Choosing a country like Ecuador or the Seychelles with low AIDS, Hepatitis and other blood-borne illnesses is vital. The mother's blood is

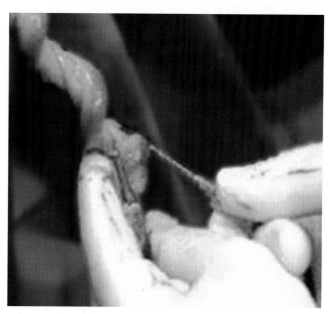

**Fig. 2.11:** Cord blood extraction

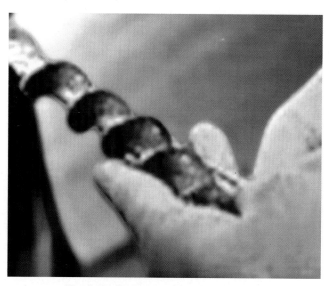

**Fig. 2.12:** Doctor extracting the cord blood

checked by an independent laboratory near the time of birth to verify noninfectious status. Newborn blood is much less likely to show markers of infectious illness, even if it showed up in maternal blood. Donated cells are never used until the laboratory declares it clear of such markers.

### Collecting Umbilical Cord Mesenchymal Stem Cells

After collection of blood, the umbilical cord is cut off from the placenta, and kept cold until it is processed. The blood vessels are removed from the cord, and the cord is cut into one centimeter sections. The cord pieces are soaked in an enzyme cocktail for an hour or so. The enzymes break down the matrix around the mesenchymal stem cells, releasing them into the fluid, which is centrifuged to settle the cells, and washed. The cells may then be expanded, stored or used.

### Separation—Gravimetric

Cord blood stem cells can be simply removed from cord blood by centrifugation **(Fig. 2.13)**. Cord blood is layered with a special fluid which is lighter slightly (less dense) than the stem cells. After centrifuging at a force about thousand times the force of gravity, stem cells are found in a layer between the blood cells and the fluid level.

### Fluorescent Marking

Stem cells of different types can also be identified by particular proteins on their membranes **(Fig. 2.14)**. Antibodies can be created to find and bind to these proteins. If the antibodies are then marked with fluorescent dyes, the characteristic identifying proteins on the cells can be seen using the fluorescent microscope or scanned with a flow cytometer.

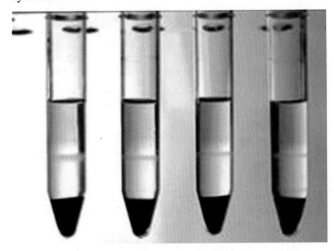

**Fig. 2.13:** Separation—Gravimetric

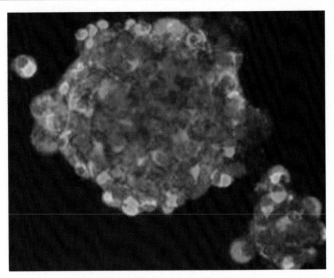

**Fig. 2.14:** Different types of stem cells

### Fluorescent Cell Separation

A flow cytometer can identity the different cell types by looking at their size, internal structure and tagged markers on the surface proteins **(Fig. 2.15)**. A special $400,000 version of flow cytometer, called a "cell sorter", can actually separate one cell type from the others.

### Magnetic Marking

Instead of dyes, the identifying proteins can be marked with tiny magnetic spheres **(Fig. 2.16)**.

### Magnetic Separation

A magnet that separates the marked and unmarked cells **(Fig. 2.17)**.

### Division of Therapies

- Phase I Therapies—Unprocessed stem cells
- Phase II Therapies—Expanded cell lines
- Phase III Therapies—Differentiated cell precursors.

### Phase I Therapies—Unprocessed Stem Cells

Pre-screened, disease-free placentae and umbilical cords are collected and the blood removed from them. Umbilical cord blood stem cells (UCB stem cells) are separated from umbilical cord blood within 24 hours.

- Using umbilical cord blood stem cells overcome the potential downside of other types of stem cell therapy
- Some stem cell types, especially embryonic stem cells, tend to degenerate and form tumors when transplanted.

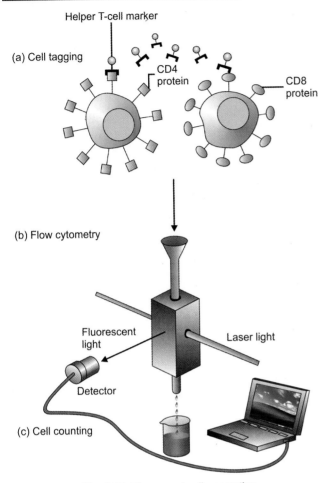

Fig. 2.15: Fluorescent cell separation

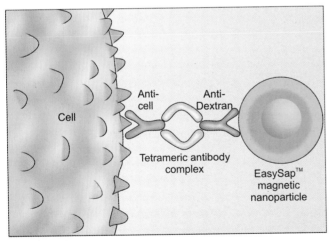

Fig. 2.16: Magnetic marking

Adult stem cells and umbilical cord stem cells do not have this tendency

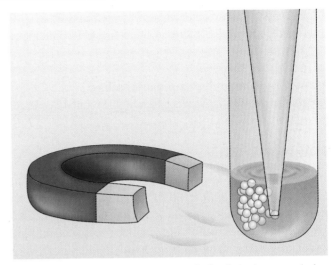

Fig. 2.17: Bead-bound molecules ready for downstream analysis

- Adult stem cells can cause immune reactions when transplanted into another person
- Rejection of the transplant or graft can happen but umbilical cord stem cells seem to lack this response
- These cells are excellent for use in anti-aging. Stem cells increase libido, energy and strength, thicken thinning skin, increase muscle and bone mass, improve heart and immune system function, increase eyesight in many cases, improve lung function in many cases
- They are also good for skin conditions, arthritis and joint problems, kidney, liver, heart and many more.

The following is a partial list of improvements reported by recipients:

- *Cardiac*: Restore cardiac function and stop arrhythmias. Repair heart muscle and blood supply. Rebuild some valves
- *Lungs*: Improve function in some cases
- *MS*: Improve many cases
- *Kidneys*: Improve many cases
- *Liver*: Improve liver function. Regrow damaged liver
- *Metabolic disease*: Cure many cases of devastating metabolic disease
- *Neurologic*: Improves memory in many cases. Reverses MS and ALS. Very effective in stroke and cerebral palsy
- *Cancer*: Improves immune system function. Repairs or replaces damaged immune system. Sometimes regrows normal tissue to replace cancer
- *Blood disorders*: Replaces damaged marrow, curing many cases

- *Diabetes*: Cures some cases of Types I and II
- *Bones and joints*: Increase bone mass. Repair many arthritic joints
- *Skin*: Skin disorders
- *Surgery*: Improved post-surgical healing
- *Endocrine gland disorders*: Renew and regulate youthful hormone levels.

### Phase II Therapies—Expanded Cell Lines

It is expected that increasing the doses of stem cells will allow greater ability to repair damaged body parts, and an increased ability to stimulate native cells to repair function. Expansion is the term for allowing stem cells to multiply and increase their numbers **(Fig. 2.18)**. The minimum dose for an adult can be found in one cord blood donation (unit). Some units are smaller, and may have only half as many stem cells. Expansion of the cells, which can double up to 10 times without a problem, ensures effective use of smaller cord blood donations. Allowing the stem cells to multiply will increase the number of stem cells transplanted, and likely increase the chance of effective treatment and healing. Still, since stem cells can multiply and produce more stem cells, and more of the needed differentiated cell type, it may not be necessary to give large amounts of stem cells. Mor e research will determine optimum numbers for different conditions. Further expansion will allow several people to be treated with only one unit of donated cord blood. Overexpansion may decrease the cell's ability to multiply

within the body, thus robbing them of some of their effectiveness.

### Phase III Therapies—Differentiated Cell Precursors

Differentiating the stem cells into the precursor cells for different cell types allows more specific targeting of cells to a specific damaged organ **(Fig. 2.19)**.

- *Nerve cell precursors*: Stroke repair, cerebral palsy, dementia, memory loss, traumatic brain injury, spinal cord injury.
- *Mesenchymal stem cells*: Kidney repair, liver repair, pancreas, brain cells, intestinal disorders, bone and joint problems.
- *Liver/Pancreas precursors*: Diabetes Types I and II, hepatitis, liver disease and liver cancer.
- *Hematopoietic stem cells*: Anemia, bone marrow disorders, immune disorders, cancer, chronic infections, lupus, rheumatoid arthritis.
- *Skin stem cells*: Burns, skin grafts, skin disorders.
- *Muscle precursor cells*: Muscular dystrophy, cardiomyopathy, heart attack damage.
- *Lung cell precursors*: Emphysema. Lung disorders.

Comparison of mature and early stem cells **(Fig. 2.20)** and their advantages and disadvantages are depicted in **Tables 2.1 and 2.2.**

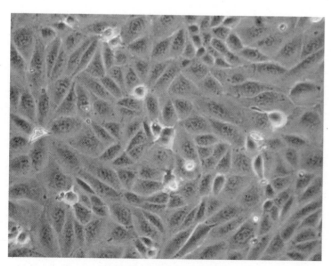

Fig. 2.18: Expanded call lines

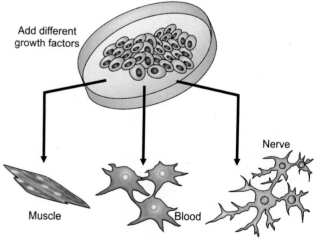

Fig. 2.19: Differentiating the stem cells into the precursor cells for all types

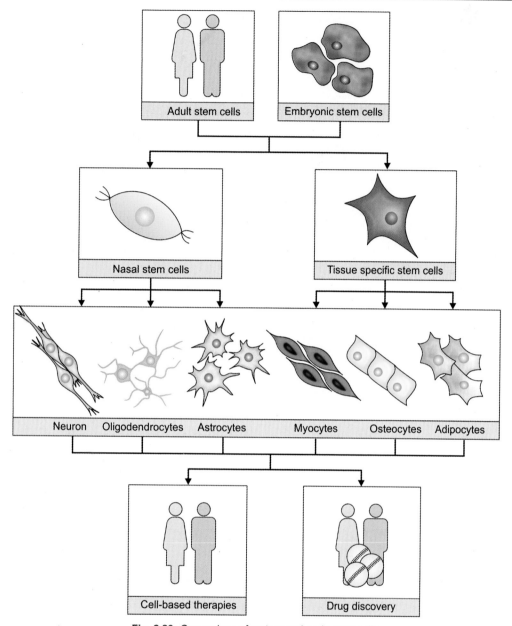

**Fig. 2.20:** Comparison of mature and early stem cells

**TABLE 2.1:** Comparison of mature and early stem cells

| *Mature stem cells aka adult, somatic* | *Early stem cells aka, embryonic, blastocystic* |
|---|---|
| • Obtained from mature body tissues, umbilical cord and placenta after birth | • Obtained from the *inner cell mass* of a blastocyst |
| • Primarily *multipotent*; give rise to limited cell types | • *Pluripotent*; give rise to all cell types (except the cells of the *placenta*) |
| • First isolated in the 1960s | • First isolated in 1998 by researchers at the *University of Wisconsin* |
| • Federal funding (FY 1999-2004): $2.248 | • Federal funding (FY 2002-2004): $55M |
| • Results: 50+ human therapies | • Results: Only in animal trials, no human trials to date |

**TABLE 2.2:** Advantages and disadvantages of mature and early stem cells

| *Mature stem cells* | |
|---|---|
| *Advantages* | *Disadvantages* |
| • Immune response is unlikely because patients are using their own cells<br>• Some availability (e.g. blood stem cells)<br>• Partly specialized; require less coaxing to create specialized cells | • Limited longevity; difficult to maintain in cell culture for long periods<br>• Difficult to find and extract from mature tissues<br>• Many unknowns; not all mature stem cell types have been identified yet<br>• Multipotent; limited flexibility; cannot become any cell type to date<br>• Uncommon and growing more scarce with age<br>• Questionable quality due to genetic defects; targeted disease may still be present in stem cell genes. |

| *Early stem cells* | |
|---|---|
| *Advantages* | *Disadvantages* |
| • Immortal; cell lines remain intact for long periods of time and produce endless numbers of cells<br>• Easy to extract in a laboratory<br>• *Pluripotent*; very flexible; can make any body cell<br>• Readily available; many blastocysts created by *in vitro* fertilization are available for research purposes; new methods like SCNT are opening up new potential sources<br>• With somatic cell nuclear transfer (SCNT), immune rejection is not an issue because the patients are using their own cells | • Immune rejection is possible if stem cells are derived from an blastocyst created through *in vitro* fertilization (IVF)<br>• Difficult to control; may require many steps to coax into desired cell type |

# CHAPTER 3

# Embryonic Stem Cells

As the name suggests, *embryonic stem cells* are derived from embryos. These embryos develop from eggs that have been fertilized *in vitro* (in an *in vitro* fertilization clinic) **(Fig. 3.1)**. It is then donated for research purposes with the informed consent of the donors. The embryos from which human embryonic stem cells are derived are typically four or five days old and are a hollow microscopic ball of cells called the *blastocyst* **(Figs 3.2 and 3.3)**. Please bear in mind that these embryos are *not* derived from eggs fertilized in a woman's body. Once formed these embryonic stem cells have the potential to produce body cells of all types.

A **blastocyst** (BLAST-oh-sist) is a preimplantation embryo that develops five days after the fertilization of an egg by a sperm. It contains all the material necessary for the development of a complete human being **(Figs 3.4 and 3.5)**.

The blastocyst includes three structures:
1. The *trophoblast* (outer cell mass) is a layer of cells that surrounds the blastocyst.
2. The *blastocoel* is a hollow cavity inside the blastocyst.
3. The *inner cell mass* (Embryoblast) is composed of approximately 30-34 cells at one end of the blastocoel. It is referred to by scientists as *pluripotent,* because they can differentiate into all of the cell types of the body.

In common usage, "embryo" refers to all stages of development, from fertilization until a somewhat ill-defined stage when it is called a fetus. Terms such as "morula" and "blastocyst" are used by scientists to refer to precise, specific stages of preimplantation development **(Fig. 3.6)**. In order to be accurate, this booklet uses scientific terms when describing scientific concepts, but uses the term "embryo" where more precision seemed likely to confuse rather than clarify.

During normal development, the blastocyst would implant itself in the endometrium uterus to become the embryo and continue to develop into a mature organism. While the outer cells would begin to form the placenta, the inner cell mass would begin to differentiate into the (which become) progressively more specialized body cell types.

## PROPERTIES

Embryonic stem (ES) cells are pluripotent, which means they are able to differentiate into all derivatives of the three primary germ layers:
1. Ectoderm
2. Endoderm
3. Mesoderm.

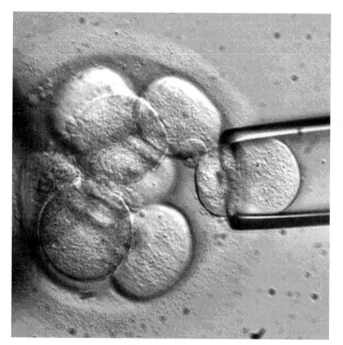

Fig. 3.1: Embryos

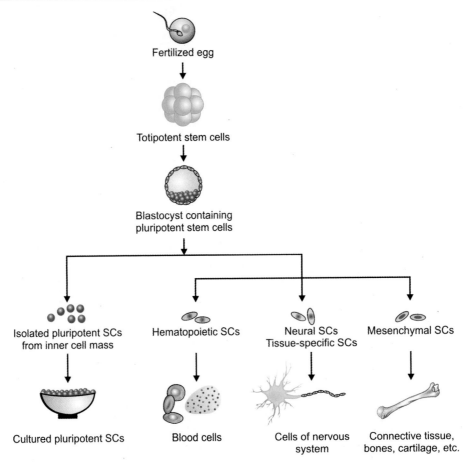

Fig. 3.2: Embryonic stem cells capable of producing many cell types

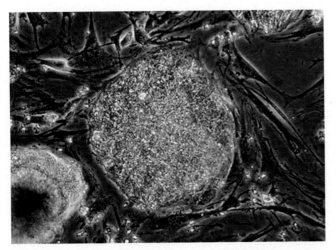

Fig. 3.3: Embryonic stem cells under the microscope

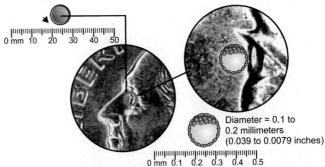

Fig. 3.4: A blastocyst is a microscopic group of cells that is small enough to fit into Roosevelt's eye on the face of a US dime

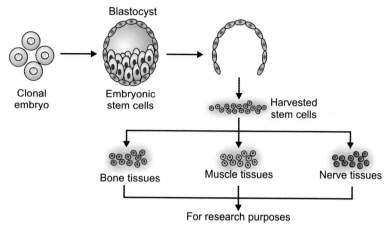

**Fig. 3.5:** Generation of embryonic stem cells

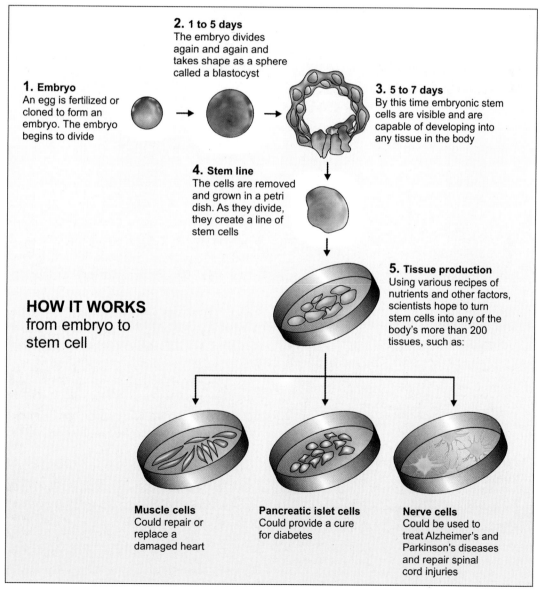

**2. 1 to 5 days**
The embryo divides
again and again and
takes shape as a sphere
called a blastocyst

**1. Embryo**
An egg is fertilized or
cloned to form an
embryo. The embryo
begins to divide

**3. 5 to 7 days**
By this time embryonic stem
cells are visible and are
capable of developing into
any tissue in the body

**4. Stem line**
The cells are removed
and grown in a petri
dish. As they divide,
they create a line of
stem cells

**5. Tissue production**
Using various recipes of
nutrients and other factors,
scientists hope to turn
stem cells into any of the
body's more than 200
tissues, such as:

**HOW IT WORKS**
from embryo to
stem cell

**Muscle cells**
Could repair or
replace a
damaged heart

**Pancreatic islet cells**
Could provide a cure
for diabetes

**Nerve cells**
Could be used to
treat Alzheimer's and
Parkinson's diseases
and repair spinal
cord injuries

**Fig. 3.6:** From embryo to stem cell; < 8 weeks—embryo; 8 weeks to till delivery—fetus

These derivatives include not less than 220 types of cells in the adult body. ES cells can be distinguished from multipotent progenitor cells by means of pluripotency. The multipotent progenitor cells, found in the adults, form only a limited number of cell types. ES cells maintain the pluripotency through multiple cell divisions, if they are not given stimuli for differentiation (i.e. when grown *in vitro*). Though the presence of pluripotent adult stem cells remains a subject of scientific debate, research has been reported to demonstrate that pluripotent stem cells can be directly generated from adult fibroblast cultures.

As depicted in the **Figure 3.7**, when the blastocyst is used for stem cell research, scientist's first remove the inner cell mass. They then place these cells in a culture dish with a nutrient-rich liquid; this in turn gives rise to embryonic stem cells. Embryonic stem cells are said to be more flexible than the stem cells found in adults (adult stem cells), because they have the potential to produce every cell type in the human body. They are easier to collect, purify and maintain in the laboratory than the adult stem cells. Scientists can induce these embryonic stem cells to replicate themselves in an undifferentiated state for very long periods of time before stimulating them to differentiate into specialized cells. This means that just a few embryonic stem cells can build a large bank of stem cells to be used in experiments. However, such undifferentiated stem cells cannot be used

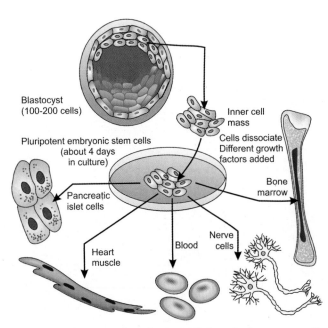

**Fig. 3.7:** Pluripotent, embryonic stem cells from the inner mass cells within a blastocyst can become any tissue in the body

directly for tissue transplants as their uncontrolled division can cause a type of tumor called *teratoma*. The embryonic stem cells would first have to be differentiated into specialized cell types before they can be used for therapies.

## FACTORS INVOLVED IN SELF-RENEWAL AND PLURIPOTENCY OF EMBRYONIC STEM CELLS

A. *Extrinsic factors*:
   1. Leukemia inhibitory factor (LIF)
   2. BMP4
   3. bFGF
   4. Other suggested factors
B. *Intrinsic factors*:
   1. Oct4
   2. Sox2
   3. Foxd3
   4. Nanog
   5. miRNA

### Extrinsic Factors Governing Maintenance of the Undifferentiated State of Embryonic Stem Cells

#### Leukemia Inhibitory Factor (LIF)

The LIF belongs to the family of interleukin-6 (IL-6)-type cytokines. The IL-6 type cytokines stimulate cells through the gp130 receptor. The gp130 works as a heterodimer together with a ligand specific receptor (such as LIF-R). While the gp130 is expressed in all cells of the body, the specific subunits are expressed in a cell-specific manner (CM). After the discovery of LIF as the active factor in CM, it was shown that the oncostatin M (OSM) and the ciliary neutrophic factor (CNF) (Conover et al. 1993), which also belong to the IL-6 cytokine family, can substitute the need for CM. Their similar effect seems to be attributed to their shared downstream effectors.

Activation of the gp130 → activation of both the Janus associated tyrosine kinase (JAK) and the signal transducer and activator of transcription (STAT) proteins → their translocation to the nucleus → binding to DNA → subsequent activation of transcription.

It has been shown that the ability of LIF to prevent differentiation of MESCs is dependent upon activation of STAT3. Concurrently, STAT3 activation even in the absence of LIF is sufficient to enable the propagation of the cells. In addition to the activation of STAT3, which is involved in the maintenance of the undifferentiated state, LIF also induces additional signals, including the activation of ERKs (extracellular receptor kinases). The activation of ERKs promotes differentiation. Thus, the balance between the activation of STAT3 and the activation of ERK signals determines the fate of the dividing undifferentiated ES cell. Therefore, signals that control the activation of ERKs also have an important role in maintaining the undifferentiated state.

Lately, it has been shown that inhibition of PI3K (phosphoinositide 3-kinase) leads to differentiation of MESCs. The PI3K signalling pathway is also induced by LIF, and the differentiation observed upon its inhibition is the result of augmented levels of activated ERKs.

An additional report suggests another pathway activated by LIF in MESCs. This pathway involves the activation of the Src family of nonreceptor tyrosine kinases, and specifically its member cYes. Inhibition of this family decreases the growth and expression of ES cell markers, both in MESCs and HESCs. The activity of cYes in MESCs is regulated both by LIF and by serum, and it is downregulated upon differentiation. However, it seems that cYes does not have a central function *in vivo*, since mice mutated in cYes are viable and fertile **(Table 3.1)**.

Human ES cells (HESCs) also require co-culture with feeders, but in human cells this requirement cannot be substituted by the addition of LIF (from human or mouse origin). Mouse LIF does not act on human cells, and therefore cannot be the protein secreted from the MEF cells that maintains HESCs pluripotency. In HESCs, just as in MESCs, the co-culture with feeders can be substituted by the addition of CM, and a prolonged feeder-free culture can be maintained in the presence of certain extracellular matrixes (like matrigel or laminin) together with CM.

When exploring the reason for the lack of responsiveness of HESCs to LIF, it was first hypothesized that this was a result of low or absent expression of LIF-R. However, when this hypothesis was examined, it was observed that a variety of LIF-R expression levels can be found in different HESC lines, ranging from low or absent to significant levels of expression. In addition, recent papers have shown that the reason for lack of LIF effect on HESCs is not the inability of the cells to respond to LIF signalling, but rather the activation of STAT3 in HESCs, which in MESCs is sufficient for self-renewal, does not prevent differentiation of HESCs. Additionally, in the undifferentiated state of HESCs, the STAT3 pathway is not activated. While in undifferentiated MESCs a high level of phosphorylated STAT3 (which is the active form) can be found, this activated form is not seen in undifferentiated HESCs.

### BMP4

BMP4, a member of the TGF-beta superfamily of polypeptide signalling molecules, was recently suggested to be involved in the prevention of MESC differentiation as well. Although LIF is sufficient to prevent MESC differentiation in the presence of serum, when serum is removed, even in the presence of LIF, neural differentiation occurs. Since serum contains many unknown factors, it seems that at least some of them prevent ES cell differentiation. Addition of BMP4 to the media enables serum-free culture. This is possible only in the presence of LIF, since otherwise differentiation to non-neural lineages takes place. Withdrawal of both BMP4 and LIF results in neural differentiation. Therefore, LIF is needed to maintain the undifferentiating capacity of BMP4, which in the absence of LIF actually drives the cells to differentiate. Thus, it seems that while BMP4 acts to prevent differentiation to neural lineages, LIF works to inhibit differentiation to non-neural lineages.

BMP4 supports self-renewal of MESCs through the activation of Smad proteins. They in turn activate Id genes, which are negative bHLH factors. MESCs with Id genes can grow in a serum-free culture in the absence of BMP4. Serum

| Protein | Mutant mice | Role in MESCs | Role in HESC maintenance |
|---------|-------------|---------------|--------------------------|
| | **TABLE 3.1:** Cytokines required for ES self-renewal | | |
| LIF | Develop to term, fertile, essential for embryo implantation (Stewart et al 1992) | Replaces the need for feeder cells. (Smith et al 1998; Williams et al 1998) | No apparent role in self-renewal (Daheron et al 2004) |
| BMP4 | Do not proceed beyond egg cylinder stage. Failure of gastrulation and mesoderm formation (Winnier et al 1995) | Replaces the need for serum presence (Ying et al 2003) | Drives HESCs to trophectoderm differentiation (Xu et al 2004) |
| bFGF | Viable with defects in neural developmentand function (Dono et al 1998) | Not required for their propagation | Required for propagationin serum replacement media (Amit et al 2000) |

was also shown to induce Id gene expression through multiple pathways, and MESCs grown in the presence of serum (with no BMP4 addition) show expression of Id genes.

In HESCs, however, the addition of BMP4 to the media does not enhance self-renewal of the cells, as was observed for the MESCs. Actually BMP4 drives the cells to differentiate to trophoblast cells. This is in contrast to MESCs, which do not seem to have the capacity to differentiate to this cell type. This difference in the abilities to create trophoblast has raised the notion that HESCs and MESCs may be derived from different stages in development, and thus their self-renewal capacity may be affected by different factors.

### bFGF

bFGF has been shown to be required for the routine culture of HESCs in the presence of serum replacement. In serum free media not substituted with bFGF, the cells differentiate, while its addition makes the cells morphology more compact and enables prolonged undifferentiated culture under these conditions. In addition, bFGF enhances the cloning efficiency of the cells. While the addition of bFGF is not required for the propagation of MESCs, it was shown to be important for different pluripotent cells, embryonic germ (EG) cells, in both human and mouse. bFGF is needed to convert the transient proliferating population of primordial germ cells to an indefinitely proliferating population of EG cells. However, in the case of mouse EG cells, once the EG cell culture is established, bFGF is no longer needed for their routine culture.

Investigations that examined the expression of different elements of signalling pathways in HESCs have shown the presence of elements of FGF signalling, including all four FGF receptors and certain components of their downstream cascade, which are enriched in undifferentiated HESCs in comparison to their differentiated derivatives. bFGF is expressed by HESCs, but apparently its level is not enough to prevent differentiation.

### Other Suggested Factors

Since neither LIF nor BMP4 support self-renewal of HESCs, the search for other factors that can replace CM in HESCs continues. Even in MESCs there is evidence of self-renewal pathways that are independent of LIF or STAT3 activation. This coincides with the observation that LIF does not seem to be fundamental for the creation of pluripotency in vivo in mouse. For these reasons, it is plausible that another physiological pathway is fundamental for both human and mouse pluripotency.

One report has implicated the Wnt pathway as able to maintain HESC self-renewal for a short period of time (**Fig. 3.8**). Another report suggested that TGFα1, in combination with fibronectin and LIF are sufficient for feeder and CM-free culture. However, neither of these protocols is used routinely to grow HESCs in feeder-independent cultures.

## Intrinsic Factors Governing Maintenance of the Undifferentiated State of Embryonic Stem Cells

### Oct4

Oct4 is a transcription factor belonging to the POU transcription factor family that possesses an octamer recognition sequence, an 8-bp sequence found in the promoters and enhancers of many ubiquitously expressed and cell-specific genes. One of the unique features of Oct4 is its expression pattern, which seems to be restricted to pluripotent lineages, although its reactivation in some cancers has been reported. It is expressed in the mouse embryo from the early stages of 4- to 8-cell stage embryos until the epiblast begins to differentiate, with expression persisting in germ cells. Mouse embryos with a mutated Oct4 die following implantation due to a lack of an ICM. The role of Oct4 in maintaining HESC pluripotency is in concordance with its role in MESCs.

The target genes of Oct4 activity and the regulators it works with are not fully identified, but this information is beginning to unravel, especially in MESCs. Based on different lines of evidence, different target genes have been suggested. The genes identified include Fgf4, the transcriptional co-factor Utf-1, the zinc finger protein Rex-, platelet-derived growth factor α receptor, osteopontin (OPN), Fbx15, and more. Oct4 has also been reported to repress several genes expressed in trophoblast, such as human chorionic gonadotropin α in human choriocarcinoma cells. The way in which the activation of Oct4 target genes establishes and maintains pluripotency is still unknown, partly because not all the targets are known or studied, and partly because the target genes that have been studied so far, did not prevent the establishment of the ICM when they were disrupted.

By combining with different co-factors, Oct4 can act both as a transcriptional activator and as a transcriptional repressor. Oct4 has few known co-factors, including the adeno virus E1A, the Sry-related factor Sox-2, Foxd3, and HMG-1. Oct4 co-factors are expressed at different expression patterns in pluripotent cells (**Table 3.2**).

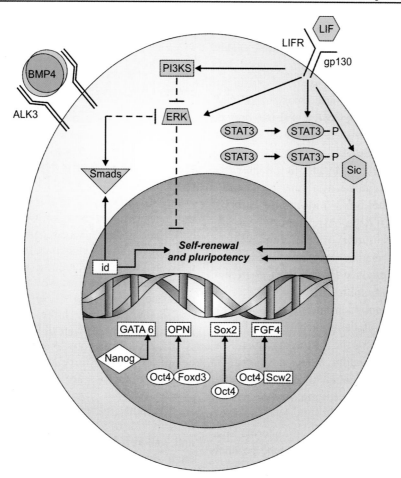

**Fig. 3.8:** Major pathways involved in mouse ES cell self-renewal

| | TABLE 3.2: Major transcription factors involved in ES self-renewal | | |
|---|---|---|---|
| *Gene* | *Mutant mice* | *Role in MESCs* | *Expression in HESCs and role in self-renewal* |
| Oct4 | Die following implantation due to lack of ICM | Required to prevent differentiation to trophoblast. Overexpression leads to differentiation to extraembryonic endoderm and ectoderm | Expressed in multiple ES cell lines. Role in self-renewal has been shown to be as inthe MESCs |
| Nanog | Consisted only of disorganized extra-embryonic tissues with no epiblast or extraembryonic ectoderm | Required to prevent differentiation to primitive endoderm Overexpression enables LIF independent growth | Expressed in multiple ES cell lines |
| Sox2 | Fail to survive shortly after implantation. Develop a normal ICM, but later lack egg cylinder structure and fail to maintain their epiblast | MESCs from null embryos cannot be established Initially their outgrowths seem normal, but later produce only trophectoderm and parietal endoderm cells | Expressed in multiple ES cell lines |
| Foxd3 | Die shortly after implantation. The size of their epiblast is reduced and the primitive streak is absent | MESCs from null embryos cannot be established, although initially their outgrowths seem normal. Have expansion of the extraembryonic ectoderm | Expressed only in some ES cell lines and therefore seems dispensable |

## Sox2

Sox2 is a member of the Sox (SRY-related HMG box) gene family that encodes transcription factors with a single HMG DNA-binding domain. Like Oct-4, it is expressed in the pluripotent lineages of the early mouse embryo, the ICM, epiblast and germ cells. But unlike Oct4, it is also expressed in the multipotential cells of the extraembryonic ectoderm and has also been shown to mark neural progenitors of the central nervous system and be important for the maintenance of their identity. Its downregulation is correlated with a commitment to differentiate. Sox2- null mouse embryos seem normal at the blastocyst stage, but fail to survive shortly after implantation. These embryos lack egg cylinder structures and lack the epithelial cells typical of the epiblast. When cultured *in vitro* to produce ES cell lines, Sox2 null blastocysts progress normally in the first days, but later do not show the normal differentiation into the ICM, and the only cells observed are trophectoderm and parietal endoderm cells. Therefore, although *in vivo* the role of Sox2 manifests by knockout only after implantation, it does have a role in maintaining the pluripotent population of cells in the earlier embryonic stages from which ES cells are derived, namely the ICM and epiblast.

Early embryos have substantial levels of maternal Sox2 protein, which unlike most of the maternal gene products persists until implantation. Even in Sox2-null embryos, maternal Sox2 protein persists until the blastocyst stage. Therefore, the reason that the mutated embryos survive until implantation may be the sufficient levels of maternal Sox2 protein until that stage. Hence, it may be that Sox2 does indeed have a role in maintaining or creating pluripotency in earlier stages, but this role cannot be detected in simple knockout experiments due to the presence of the maternal protein. In addition, Sox2 also has a role in the maintenance of trophoblast stem cells, and in the absence of Sox2 these cells cannot be generated.

## Foxd3

Foxd3 (originally called genesis) belongs to the fork head family genes. It is not expressed in unfertilized oocytes or one cell stage fertilized embryos, but its transcripts are detected in blastocyst stage embryos. Foxd3- null embryos die around the time of gastrulation with a loss of the epiblast and an expansion of extraembryonic ectoderm and endoderm. However, in the blastocyst stage their ICM appears normal, with normal expression of ICM markers **(Fig. 3.9)**. When cultured *in vitro*, Foxd3-null blastocysts seem normal initially, but later their ICM fails to expand. Chimeric rescue experiments have shown that Foxd3-null cells are able to differentiate into many cell types. Thus, it seems that Foxd3 may be required for the regulation of either a secreted factor or a cell-surface signalling molecule.

## Nanog

An additional gene recently described as involved in self-renewal of ES cells is Nanog. Nanog is a homeobox transcription factor, which does not belong to any known group of homeobox genes. It is expressed in the mouse in the inner cells of the compacted morula and blastocyst, early germ cells, ES cells, embryonic germ cells (EGs), and embryonic carcinoma cells (ECs), and is absent from differentiated cells. Nanog was named after the mythological Celtic land of the ever young, Tir Nanog, since over-expression of Nanog in MESCs renders the cells independent of LIF supply. Although the cells self-renewal and remain pluripotent in the absence of LIF, their self-renewal capacity is reduced. Therefore, Nanog overexpression does not completely relieve the cells from LIF dependence, but when these two factors are combined, they work together synergistically.

The Nanog overexpression effect is not mediated through the activation of STAT3, and *vice versa*, and therefore STAT3 and Nanog pathways would seem to act independently of each other. Nanog overexpressing cells can also be propagated in serum-free media in the absence of BMP, and it appears that the overexpression of Nanog maintains a substantial constitutive level of Id expression. However, Nanog overexpression does not overcome the need for Oct4 activity, and both Nanog and Oct4 are required for MESC self-renewal. Nanog disruption in MESCs results in differentiation to extraembryonic endoderm lineages.

Therefore, Nanog is essential for the maintenance of pluripotency of the ICM at one stage later than the initial requirement for Oct4. Consequently, if Oct4 operates to inhibit the differentiation of ES cells to trophoblast, Nanog works to inhibit the transition of the cells to primitive endoderm, which is the next cell fate decision in the embryo. Nevertheless, unlike Oct4 whose primary role is to prevent differentiation (to trophectoderm), Nanog not only prevents differentiation (to extraembryonic endoderm) but also actively works to maintain pluripotency. The target genes that Nanog works to activate or repress are still unknown. Nonetheless, the DNA sequence that it binds has been identified using SELEX, and target genes have been suggested based on the presence of this sequence upstream to their transcription initiation site.

One such gene is GATA6, and it seems that Nanog may repress its expression, since forced expression of GATA6

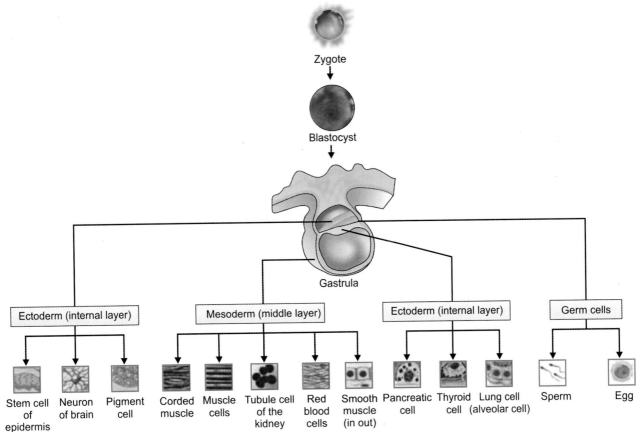

**Fig. 3.9:** Stem cell hierarchy: zygote and early cell division stages

is sufficient for differentiation to extraembryonic endoderm, the same phenotype observed in Nanog-null cells. However, Nanog also contains two domains capable of activating transcription (Pan and Pei 2004) and therefore might also positively regulate ES specific genes, on top of repressing extraembryonic endoderm genes. Human Nanog is expressed in HESCs, EC and EG cells, germ cells, and in several tumors. When human Nanog was over expressed in MESCs, partial release from LIF dependency was observed. This may indicate that the Nanog pathway in human and mouse share functional homology, but this issue is yet to be examined.

### miRNA

MicroRNAs (miRNAs) are additional regulators suggested to be involved in maintaining ES cell identity. These short RNA molecules are known to be involved in translational regulation, mostly by repressing translation and in some cases by directing miRNA to degradation.

## SOURCES OF EMBRYONIC STEM CELLS

### In Vitro Fertilization

The largest potential source of blastocysts for the research of stem cells is from *in vitro* fertilization (IVF) clinics **(Fig. 3.10)**. The process of IVF first requires the retrieval of a woman's ova. This is done via a surgical procedure after the woman has undergone an intensive regimen of "fertility drugs", which would stimulate her ovaries to produce multiple mature ova. Doctors typically fertilize all of the donated ova, when IVF is used for reproductive purposes, in order to maximize their chance of producing a viable blastocyst that can be implanted in the womb. All fertilized eggs are not implanted; this has resulted in a large bank of "excess" blastocysts that are currently stored in freezers across the country. These blastocysts can prove to be a major source of embryonic stem cells for use in medical research **(Fig. 3.11)**.

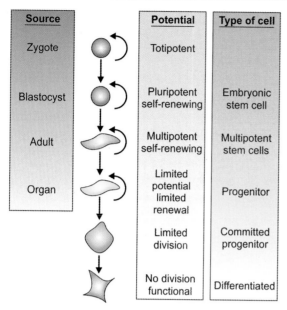

Fig. 3.10: Largest source of stem cells

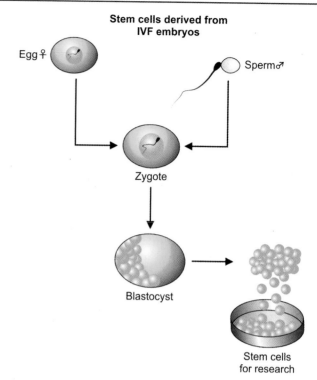

Fig. 3.11: Stem cells derived from IVF embryos

The IVF technique may also potentially be used to produce blastocysts specifically for research purposes. This would mean isolating stem cells with specific genetic traits necessary for the study of particular diseases **(Fig. 3.12)**. For example, it may be possible to study the origins of an inherited disease like cystic fibrosis using stem cells made from egg and sperm donors who have this disease.

*In vitro* differentiation of ES cells has been used in basic science to study gene expression during development of specific cell types, in addition to its clinical application. Since gene modulation techniques, including gene targeting, are well established in ES cells, it is relatively easy to identify a role of a specific gene in the development of a certain cell lineage. Further, in combination with the techniques to purify tissue-specific cells described above, we can determine the function of genes in a specific tissue solely by *in vitro* assay.

## Nuclear Transfer

This process offers another potential way to produce embryonic stem cells. Nuclear transfer, in animals, has been accomplished by inserting the nucleus of an already differentiated adult cell into a donated egg that has had its nucleus removed, for example, a skin cell **(Fig. 3.13)**. This egg now contains the genetic material of the skin cell. It is then stimulated to form a blastocyst from which the embryonic stem cells can be derived. The stem cells created in this way are copies or "clones" of the original adult cell, because their nuclear DNA matches that of the adult cell.

The embryonic stem cells created by nuclear transfer would be genetically matched to a person needing a transplant. This would make it far less likely for the patient's body to reject the new cells than it would be with traditional tissue transplant procedures. Using nuclear transfer to produce stem cells is not the same as reproductive cloning; but some are concerned about the potential misapplication of the technique for reproductive cloning purposes.

## Therapeutic Cloning

The same procedure used to clone whole organisms, such as Dolly the sheep can also be used to create ESCs. The process is called so, because of its potential medical uses **(Figs 3.14 to 3.18)**.

## EMBRYONIC STEM CELL LINES

Growing cells in the laboratory is known as cell culture. Embryonic stem cell lines (ES cell lines) are cultures of cells are derived from the epiblast tissue of the inner cell mass (ICM) of a blastocyst/earlier morula stage embryos **(Fig. 3.19)**. They are established from embryos shortly after fertilization.

An embryo must be separated into individual cells, to create an embryonic stem cell line.

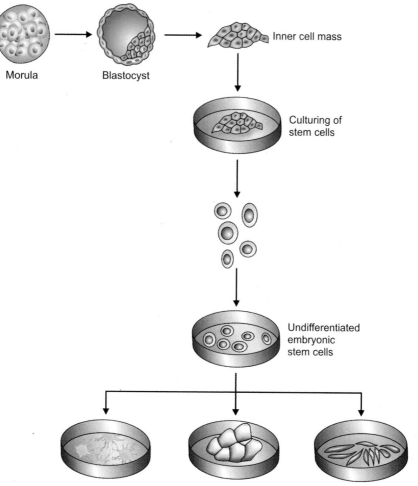

**Fig. 3.12:** Isolation and culture of human ESCs from blastocyst

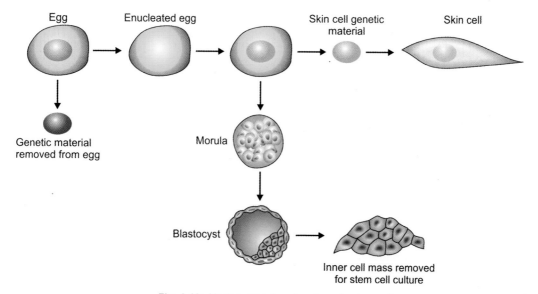

**Fig. 3.13:** Nuclear transfer of embryonic stem cell

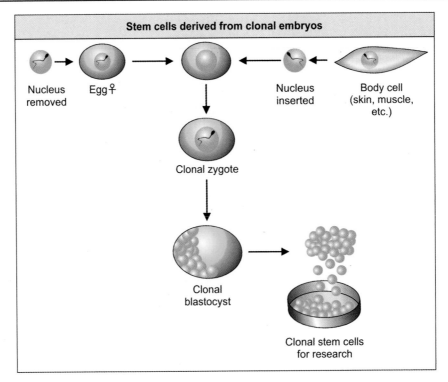

**Fig. 3.14:** Therapeutic cloning

## Procedure

Human embryonic stem cells (HESCs) are first isolated. For this the inner cell mass is transferred into a plastic laboratory culture dish that contains a nutrient broth known as culture medium. These cells divide and spread over the surface of the dish.

Typically, the inner surface of the culture dish is coated with mouse embryonic skin cells. This coating layer of cells is called a *feeder layer* and being treated, they will not divide. The feeder layer gives the ICM cells a sticky surface to which they can attach. Also, they release nutrients into the culture medium.

Over the course of several days, the cells of the inner cell mass proliferate and begin to crowd the culture dish. They are then gently removed and plated into several fresh culture dishes. The process of replanting the cells is repeated many times, for many months, and is called *subculturing*. Each cycle of subculturing the cells is referred to as a *passage*.

After six months or more, the original 30 cells of the ICM would have produced millions of ESCs. Such ESCs that have proliferated in cell culture for six months or more without differentiating, are pluripotent, and appear genetically normal are referred to as an ***embryonic stem cell line*** **(Figs 3.20 and 3.21)**.

Scientists are currently working to devise ways of growing embryonic stem cells without the mouse feeder cells, because of the risk that viruses or other macromolecules in the mouse cells may be transmitted to the human cells.

## TESTS TO IDENTIFY EMBRYONIC STEM CELLS

- Growing and subculturing the stem cells for many months, ensures that the cells are capable of long-term self-renewal. Scientists repeatedly inspect the cultures through a microscope to ascertain that the cells look healthy and remain undifferentiated
- Using specific techniques to determine the presence of surface markers, found only on undifferentiated cells. Another important test is for the presence of a protein called Oct-4, which undifferentiated cells typically make. Oct-4 is a transcription factor, it helps turn genes on and off at the right time. This is an important part of the processes of cell differentiation and embryonic development
- Examining the chromosomes under a microscope. This is done in order to assess whether the chromosomes are damaged or if the number of chromosomes has changed. However, it does not detect genetic mutations in the cells

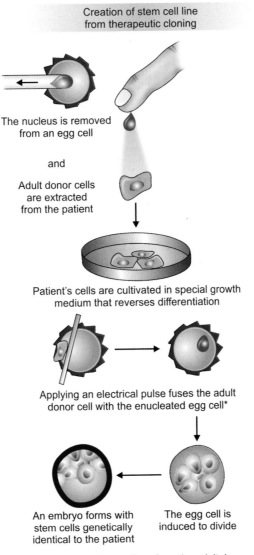

Creation of stem cell line
from therapeutic cloning

The nucleus is removed
from an egg cell

and

Adult donor cells
are extracted
from the patient

Patient's cells are cultivated in special growth
medium that reverses differentiation

Applying an electrical pulse fuses the adult
donor cell with the enucleated egg cell*

An embryo forms with          The egg cell is
stem cells genetically         induced to divide
identical to the patient

* Alternatively, the nucleus from the adult donor
cell could be directly injected into the egg cell

**Fig. 3.15:** Therapeutic cloning might be a viable approach to growing an exact tissue match for a patient in need—if the donor nucleus came from the patient, the resulting embryonic stem cell line would be a perfect match

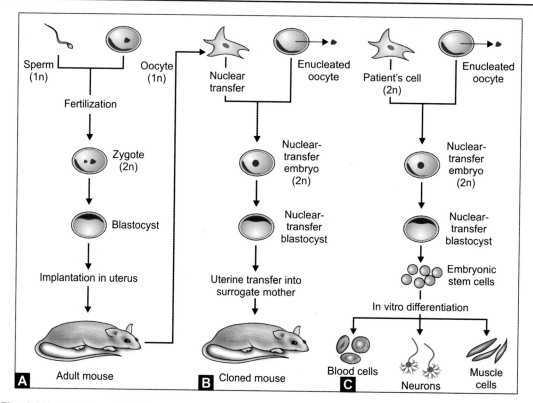

**Figs 3.16A to C:** Normal development versus development during reproductive cloning and therapeutic cloning

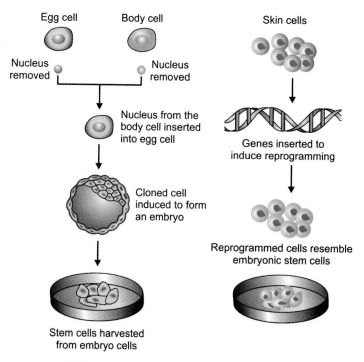

**Fig. 3.17:** Therapeutic cloning and nuclear reprogramming

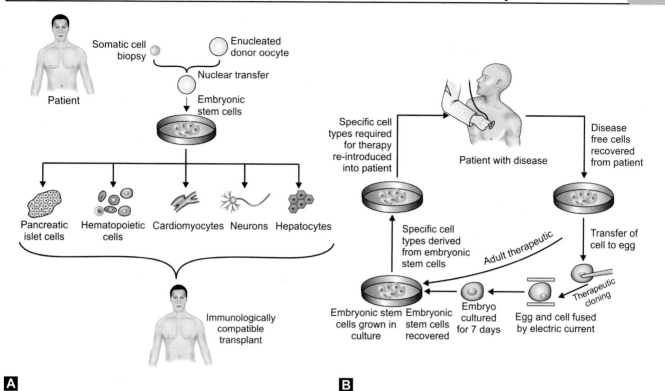

**Figs 3.18A and B:** Human therapeutic cloning

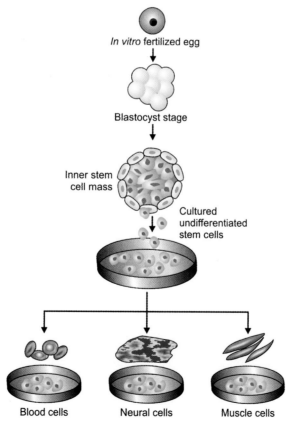

**Fig. 3.19:** ESCs obtained from epiblast tissue

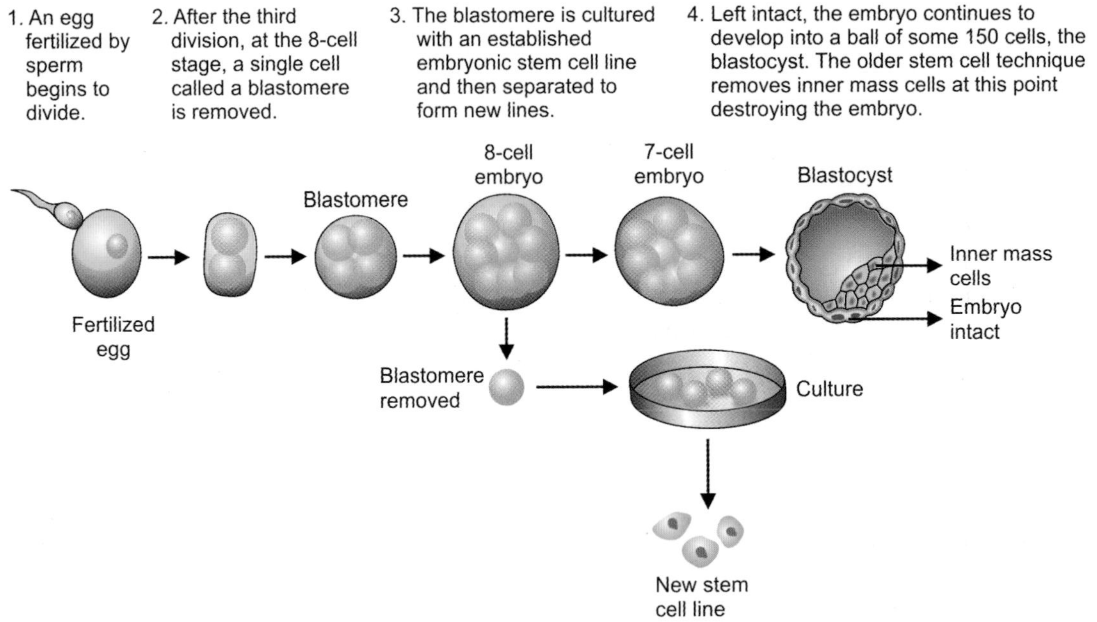

1. An egg fertilized by sperm begins to divide.

2. After the third division, at the 8-cell stage, a single cell called a blastomere is removed.

3. The blastomere is cultured with an established embryonic stem cell line and then separated to form new lines.

4. Left intact, the embryo continues to develop into a ball of some 150 cells, the blastocyst. The older stem cell technique removes inner mass cells at this point destroying the embryo.

8-cell embryo

7-cell embryo

Blastocyst

Blastomere

Fertilized egg

Inner mass cells

Embryo intact

Blastomere removed

Culture

New stem cell line

**Fig. 3.20:** One stem cell line, one growing embryo: Scientists report a new method to make human embryonic stem cells that does not, as before, destroy the embryo

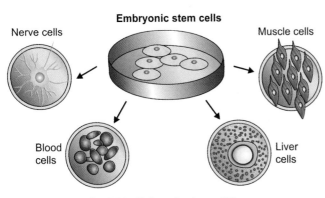

**Embryonic stem cells**

Nerve cells

Muscle cells

Blood cells

Liver cells

**Fig. 3.21:** Embryonic stem cell line

- Determining whether the cells can be subcultured after freezing, thawing and replanting
- Testing whether the HESC are pluripotent by:
  1. Allowing the cells to differentiate spontaneously in cell culture
  2. Manipulating the cells so that they will differentiate to form specific cell types
  3. Injecting the cells into an immunosuppressed mouse to test for the formation of a benign tumor called a *teratoma*.

Teratomas typically contain a mixture of many differentiated or partly differentiated cell types. This is an indication that the ESCs are capable of differentiating into multiple cell types.

## OBSTACLES AND RISKS ASSOCIATED WITH THE USE OF ESCs

It is necessary to identify and minimize, or eliminate, the risks that ESCs might pose, in addition to demonstrating the functional effectiveness of ESC transplants. Two identifiable risks:

1. Tumor formation
2. Immune rejection.

As noted earlier, HESCs injected into mice can produce a benign tumor made up of diverse tissues; this response is believed to be related to the multipotency of the undifferentiated cells in an *in vivo* environment. However, in a small number of short-term studies in mice, HESCs that have been allowed to begin the process of differentiation before transplantation have not resulted in significant tumor formation. Obviously, this is a critical problem to understand and control.

Therefore, it is too early to tell, whether it will be appropriate to use HESCs directly in regenerative medicine. A great deal obviously must be elucidated about how the body controls the differentiation of stem cells and this has yet to be reliably reproduced *in vitro*. The behavior of ESCs implanted in a specific organ also has not been studied well. It might someday be possible to add growth factors with a transplant to stimulate the production of a particular cell type or multiple cell types. "Inducer tissues" that interact with stem cells might be co-transplanted with ESCs to achieve a similar result. These possibilities are still in experimental investigation.

In another respect, the possible problems associated with ESC transplantation are common to all transplantation, such as:

• The risk of infection
• The risk of tissue rejection.

Rejection is a serious obstacle to successful transplantation of stem cells and tissues derived from them. Though it has been suggested that ESCs provoke less of an immune reaction than a whole organ transplant, it is unclear whether that will be true of the regenerated tissues derived from ESCs. Some cell types (such as dendritic cells, immune system cells, and vascular endothelial cells) carry more of the histocompatibility antigens that provoke immune reactions than other cells. These types are present in the tissues of whole organs, they connect an organ with the bloodstream and nervous system.

However, tissue derived *in vitro* from ESCs, such as liver tissue, would not contain such cells. It would theoretically trigger a milder immune response; this assumes that techniques for controlling differentiation of ESCs will be available. In addition, the liver cells would not be devoid of all surface antigens, and so, in the absence of other techniques to reduce transplant rejection, the use of immuno-suppressive drugs will still have to be used, with attendant risks of infection and toxicity **(Fig. 3.22)**.

Although difficult to conceive, the creation of a very large number of ESC lines might be one way to obtain a diversity of cells that could theoretically increase the chances of matching the histocompatibility antigens of a transplant recipient. It has further been suggested that ESCs could be made less reactive

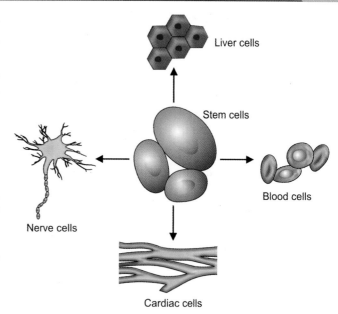

**Fig. 3.22:** Tissue derived *in vitro* from ESCs

by using genetic engineering to eliminate or introduce the presence of surface antigens on them. An exact genetic match between a transplant recipient and tissue generated from ESCs could also, in theory, be achieved by using somatic cell nuclear transfer to create histocompatible ESCs. Cells created with this technique would overcome the problem of immune rejection. However, it might to not be appropriate to transplant such cells in a person with a genetically based disease, since the cells would carry the same genetic information. In any case, an understanding of how to prevent rejection of transplanted cells is fundamental to their becoming useful for regenerative medicine and represents one of the greatest challenges for research in this field.

# Adult Stem Cells

## DEFINITION

An adult stem cell is an undifferentiated cell found among differentiated cells in a tissue or organ, can renew itself, and can differentiate to yield the major specialized cell types of the tissue or organ. The primary roles of adult stem cells in a living organism are to maintain and repair the tissue in which they are found. Some scientists now use the term somatic stem cell instead of adult stem cell. Unlike embryonic stem cells, which are defined by their origin (the inner cell mass of the blastocyst), the origin of adult stem cells in mature tissues is unknown.

Pluripotent adult stem cells are rare and generally small in number but can be found in a number of tissues including umbilical cord blood. Most adult stem cells are lineage-restricted (multipotent) and are generally referred to by their tissue origin (mesenchymal stem cell, adipose-derived stem cell, endothelial stem cell, etc.).

## HISTORY

The history of research on adult stem cells began about 40 years ago. In the 1960s, researchers discovered that the bone marrow contains at least two kinds of stem cells. One population, called hematopoietic stem cells, forms all the types of blood cells in the body. A second population, called bone marrow stromal cells, was discovered a few years later. Stromal cells are a mixed cell population that generates bone, cartilage, fat, and fibrous connective tissue **(Fig. 4.1)**.

## PROPERTIES

Unlike embryonic stem cells, adult stem cells are already somewhat specialized. For example, blood stem cells normally only give rise to the many types of blood cells, and nerve stem cells can only make the various types of

Day 28 noninduced    Day 28 induced

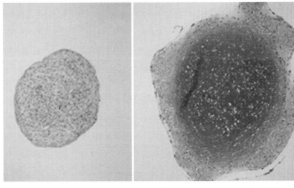

**Fig. 4.1:** *In vitro* chondrogenesis of human bone marrow derived stem cells. Three-dimensional cell pellets were cultured for 28 days in media with or without TGF-β3 supplementation (10 ng/ml). Cell pellets were embedded in paraffin, sectioned and stained with safranin O to localize the presence of proteoglycans (Red). (10 × magnification)

brain cells. Recent research however, suggests that some adult stem cells might be more flexible than previously thought, and may be made to produce a wider variety of cell types. For example, some experiments have suggested that blood stem cells isolated from adult mice may also be able to produce liver, muscle, and skin cells, but these results are not yet proven and have not been demonstrated with human cells.

Adult stem cells are often relatively slow-cycling cells able to respond to specific environmental signals and either generate new stem cells or select a particular differentiation program. When stem cell undergoes a commitment to differentiate, it often first enters a transient state of rapid proliferation. Upon exhaustion of its proliferative potential, the transiently amplifying cell withdraws from its cycle and executes its terminal differentiation program. Adult stem cells are often localized to specific niches, where they utilize many but not necessarily all, of the external and intrinsic cues used by their embryonic counterparts in selecting a specific fate.

## SOURCES OF ADULT STEM CELLS

Adult stem cells are hidden deep within organs, surrounded by millions of ordinary cells, and may help replenish some of the body's cells when needed. In fact, some adult stem cells are currently being used in therapies **(Figs 4.2 and 4.3)**. One important point to understand about adult stem cells is that there are a very small number of stem cells in each tissue. Stem cells are thought to reside in a specific area of each tissue where they may remain quiescent (nondividing) for many years until they are activated by disease or tissue injury. The adult tissues reported to contain stem cells include brain, bone marrow, peripheral blood, blood vessels, skeletal muscle, skin and liver.

## TESTS TO IDENTIFY ADULT STEM CELLS

Scientists do not agree on the criteria that should be used to identify and test adult stem cells **(Fig. 4.4)**. However, they often use one or more of the following three methods:

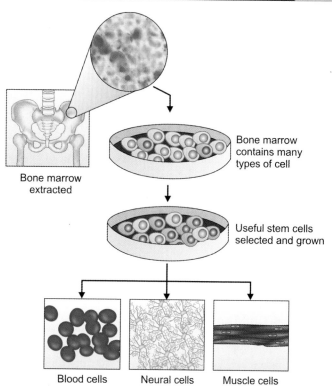

Fig. 4.3: Adult stem cells

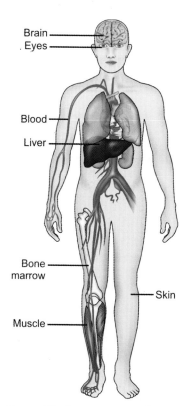

Fig. 4.2: Some of the known sources of adult stem cells

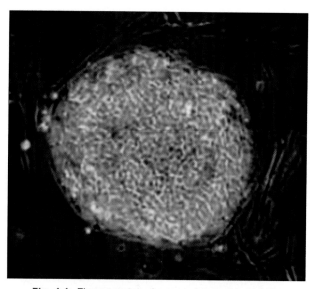

Fig. 4.4: Fluorescent markers can be used to identify stem cells among ordinary adult cells

1. Labeling the cells in a living tissue with molecular markers and then determining the specialized cell types they generate.
2. Removing the cells from a living animal, labeling them in cell culture, and transplanting them back into another animal to determine whether the cells repopulate their tissue of origin.

3. Isolating the cells, growing them in cell culture, and manipulating them, often by adding growth factors or introducing new genes, to determine what differentiated cells types they can become.

Also, a single adult stem cell should be able to generate a line of genetically identical cells known as a clone which then gives rise to all the appropriate differentiated cell types of the tissue. Scientists tend to show either that a stem cell can give rise to a clone of cells in cell culture, or that a purified population of candidate stem cells can repopulate the tissue after transplant into an animal. Recently, by infecting adult stem cells with a virus that gives a unique identifier to each individual cell, scientists have been able to demonstrate that individual adult stem cell clones have the ability to repopulate injured tissues in a living animal.

## ADULT STEM CELL DIFFERENTIATION

### Normal Differentiation Pathways of Adult Stem Cells

In a living animal, adult stem cells can divide for a long period and can give rise to mature cell types that have characteristic shapes and specialized structures and functions of a particular tissue. The following are examples of differentiation pathways of adult stem cells (**Figs 4.5 and 4.6**).

- Hematopoietic stem cells give rise to all the types of blood cells: red blood cells, B lymphocytes, T lymphocytes, natural killer cells, neutrophils, basophils, eosinophils, monocytes, macrophages, and platelets.
- Bone marrow stromal cells (mesenchymal stem cells) give rise to a variety of cell types: bone cells (osteocytes), cartilage cells (chondrocytes), fat cells (adipocytes), and other kinds of connective tissue cells such as those in tendons.
- Neural stem cells in the brain give rise to its three major cell types: nerve cells (neurons) and two categories of non-neuronal cells astrocytes and oligodendrocytes.
- Epithelial stem cells in the lining of the digestive tract occur in deep crypts and give rise to several cell types: absorptive cells, goblet cells, Paneth cells, and entero-endocrine cells.
- Skin stem cells occur in the basal layer of the epidermis and at the base of hair follicles. The epidermal stem cells give rise to keratinocytes, which migrate to the surface of the skin and form a protective layer. The follicular stem cells can give rise to both the hair follicle and to the epidermis.

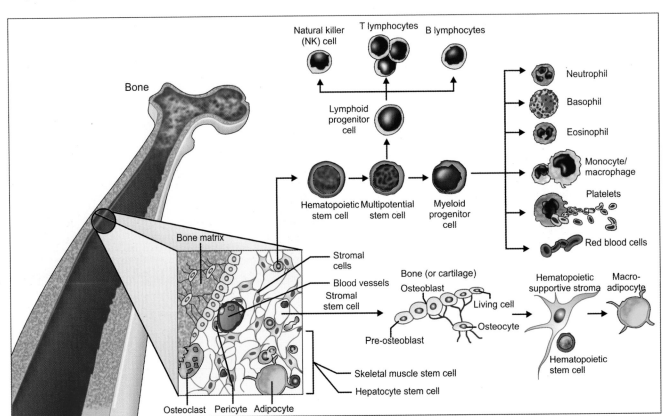

**Fig. 4.5:** Hematopoietic and stromal stem cell differentiation

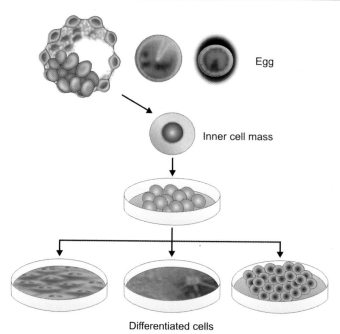

**Fig. 4.6:** Cloning with differentiated cells

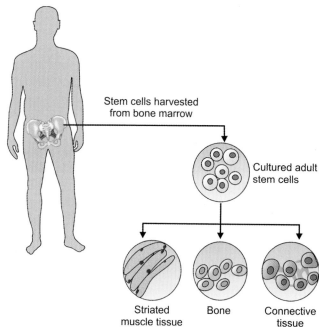

**Fig. 4.7:** Bone marrow stem cells

## ADULT STEM CELL PLASTICITY AND TRANSDIFFERENTIATION

A number of experiments have suggested that certain adult stem cell types are pluripotent. This ability to differentiate into multiple cell types is called plasticity or trans-differentiation.

## STEM CELL PLASTICITY

**Plasticity** is defined as the ability of a stem cell isolated from one tissue to "convert" to cells found in a different tissue, and sometimes even into cell types that originated from a completely different embryonic germ layer. True plasticity can be demonstrated only by the ability of a single (clonogenic) cell to form cells of multiple different pheno-types and to be shown to function as those different cell types. Recent reports of adult stem cell "plasticity" have generated a great deal of enthusiasm, as well as skepticism.The following list offers examples of adult stem cell plasticity that have been reported during the past few years:

- Hematopoietic stem cells may differentiate into: three major types of brain cells (neurons, oligodendrocytes, and astrocytes); skeletal muscle cells; cardiac muscle cells; and liver cells
- Bone marrow stromal cells may differentiate into: cardiac muscle cells and skeletal muscle cells **(Fig. 4.7)**

- Brainstem cells may differentiate into: blood cells and skeletal muscle cells.

## Pathways of Stem Cell Plasticity

Physiologic, *in vivo* expressions of differentiative potential can be seen in four flexibly employed processes or pathways.

1. First, of course, is the classic hierarchical, unidirectional concept of lineage commitment. In embryonic/fetal development, this begins with an embryonic stem cell or with a fetal stem cell. In adults, one is speaking of normative, tissue maintenance or repair after injury. In all these cases, one begins with a multi- or totipotent stem cell which, through asymmetric division, self-renews and also gives rise to more differentiated cell types. These more differentiated daughter cells mature in an ordered, hierarchical, unidirectional fashion. This model is certainly the dominant pathway for development and tissue maintenance, if not, perhaps the only pathway.

2. The second pathway of plasticity is one of "dedifferen-tiation", i.e. reversion of a differentiated cell into a pro-genitor, often blast-like (i.e. primitive or undifferentiated) phenotype, which can then give rise to different lineages. In mammals, this has only been confidently recognized in neoplasia, in particular in malignancy, in the context of genetic mutations and other genomic derangements.

3. The third is that of cells from one lineage directly differentiating into cells of another lineage. This has often

been referred to as "transdifferentiation", a term which engenders still more unnecessary debate and we now feel is best avoided. Such direct differentiative events which jump between (dogmatically) hypothesized lineage or organ boundaries have now been convincingly demonstrated *in vivo* and *ex vivo* and are induced by local microenvironmental effects that lead to alterations in gene expression.

4. The fourth pathway is that of cell-cell fusion, sometimes followed by nuclear-nuclear fusion. The idea of cell fusion was originally suggested as part of a critique of the findings regarding plasticity arising from direct differentiation, used to polemically dismiss those new findings as "artifact". However, it is now not merely a rhetorical or theoretical challenge for undermining one set of new, controversial findings, but is, itself, established as yet another alternate and surprising physiologic, *in vivo* process. In this case, the plasticity of gene expression is induced not by microenvironmental effects, but by cytoplasmic and/or nuclear factors **(Fig. 4.8)**.

## ADULT STEM CELL LINES

Adult stem cell lines isolated from mature tissues are another excellent resource for research studies. Most research is performed using adult stem cell lines from model organisms such as mice and rats, since obtaining adult stem cells from humans can involve invasive surgical procedures **(Fig. 4.9)**.

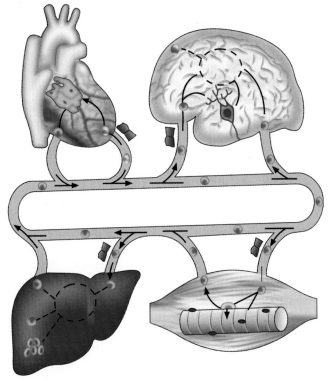

**Fig. 4.8:** Stem cell plasticity

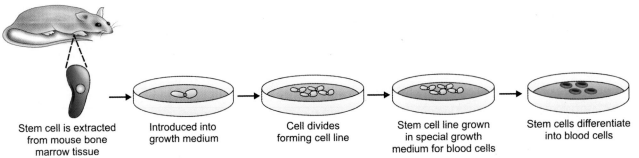

Stem cell is extracted from mouse bone marrow tissue

Introduced into growth medium

Cell divides forming cell line

Stem cell line grown in special growth medium for blood cells

Stem cells differentiate into blood cells

**Fig. 4.9:** Creation of stem cell lines from adult tissue

## Hematopoietic Adult Stem Cells

HSCs are among the few stem cells to be isolated in adult humans. They reside in the bone marrow and under some conditions migrate to other tissues through the blood. HSCs are also normally found in the fetal liver and spleen and in umbilical cord and placenta blood.

The first experimental evidence to indicate the existence of HSCs was the discovery in 1961 by Till and McCulloch of a population of clonogenic bone marrow cells capable of generating myeloerythroid colonies in the spleen of lethally irradiated hosts. Occasionally these colonies contained clonogenic cells that could be further retransplanted into secondary lethally irradiated hosts and reconstitute the immune system. These were proposed to be HSCs, i.e. progenitor cells with the essential characteristic of self-renewal and differentiation potential for all types of blood cells.

The development of clonal assays for all major hematopoietic lineages together with the availability of multi-parameter fluorescence-activated cell sorting (FACS) has enabled the prospective purification of HSCs from mice and to highly enrich for HSCs from humans according to the cell surface expression of specific molecules and their functional read-out *in vivo* and *in vitro* in stromal long-term colony initiating assays. After the identification and prospective isolation of murine HSCs, considerable progress has been made toward the characterization of the mechanisms controlling their fates. During or after cell division, the two daughter cells of a stem cell each have to decide their fate. They can either choose to remain as HSCs, commit to differentiation, or die by apoptosis and also to stay in the bone marrow or migrate to the periphery. These processes of cell-fate decisions must be finely tuned to maintain a steady-state level of functional HSCs in the bone marrow and to constantly provide progenitors for the various hematopoietic lineages **(Figs 4.10 and 4.11)**.

### *Plasticity of Hematopoietic Stem Cell (HSC)*

There is a growing body of evidence that HSCs are plastic that, at least under some circumstances, they are able to participate in the generation of tissues other than those of the blood system. A few studies have shown that HSCs can give rise to liver cells. Those findings have scientists speculating about the biological response of HSCs to disease or tissue damage and about the early differentiation of the embryonic

tissues into discrete layers **(Fig. 4.12)**. It was unexpected that a component of blood could crossover a developmental separation to form a tissue type that ordinarily has a completely different embryonic origin. The findings noted above and other reports of cardiac and muscle tissue formation after bone marrow transplantation in mice and of the development of neuron-like cells from bone marrow have raised expectations that HSCs will eventually be shown to be able to give rise to multiple cell types from all three germ layers. One study has, in fact, demonstrated that a single HSC transplanted into an irradiated mouse generated not only blood components (from the mesoderm layer of the embryo), but also epithelial cells in the lungs, gut, (endoderm layer) and skin (ectoderm layer). If HSCs are truly multipotent, their potential for life-saving regenerative therapies may be considerably expanded in the future **(Fig. 4.13)**.

## Neural Stem Cells

The discovery that stem cells exist in the adult brain was quite unexpected and required years of investigation to become widely accepted. Neural stem cells may be multipotent: when injected into blastocysts of mice they contributed to multiple types of tissues in the embryos **(Fig. 4.14)**. It was long thought that damage to the brain could not be repaired, as adult neurons could not be replaced.

A series of studies in rats and in songbirds first revealed that neurons from adult brains could be formed anew

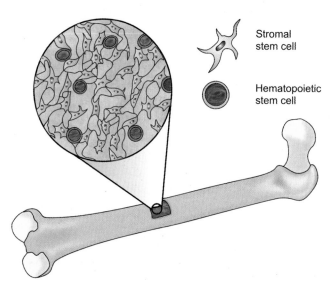

**Fig. 4.10:** Mature stem cells

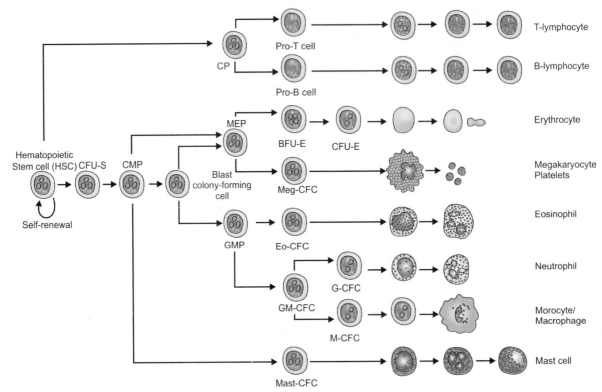

**Fig. 4.11:** The conventional view of hematopoiesis in which multipotential stem cells are self-generating and also produce precursor cells with increasing restriction of their lineage and proliferative potential. Within each lineage, population cell numbers rise with increasing maturity

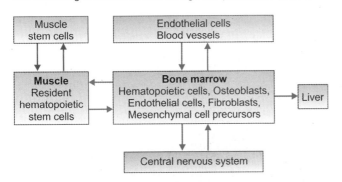

**Fig. 4.12:** Possible pathways for differentiation in adult stem cells

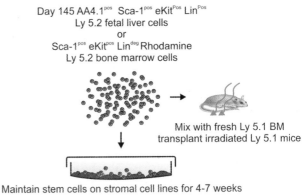

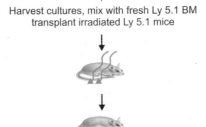

At time intervals analyze for Ly 5.2 cells in peripheral blood lineages

**Fig. 4.13:** Competitive repopulation by hematopoietic stem cells cultured with stromal cell lines

(**Fig. 4.15**). Additional studies by a number of investigators have now confirmed that mammalian adult neuronal progenitors exist and are capable of extensive cell division and self-renewal. Moreover, neural progenitors can migrate and home to specific sites of damage or regeneration, for instance to the olfactory bulb of rodents, the hippocampus of humans, and sites of tumors such as gliomas.

Thus, stem cells from the CNS provide a second source of well-characterized tissue-specific stem cells. In tissue culture and following direct injection into brains, clones from the NSC population give rise to all three major cell types of the CNS: neurons, astrocytes, and oligodendro-

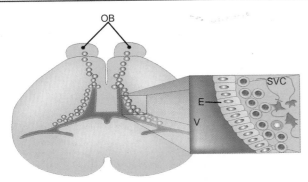

**Fig. 4.14:** Neural stem cells

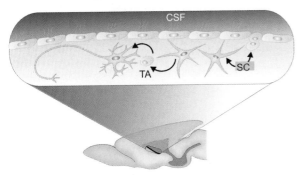

**Fig. 4.15:** In the brain, a major site of neurogenesis in adulthood appears to be close to the ventricles. In mice, the ciliated ependymal cells may serve as stem cells (*SC*), but in humans, astrocytes located in the subventricular zone (*SVZ*) have been proposed as stem cells

cytes. Following proteolytic dissociation of adult brain tissue, populations enriched for neural stem cells (NSCs) can be obtained based on differential density in a sedimentation gradient. These NSC progeny have typical morphologies, characteristic patterns of protein expression, and exhibit physiological evidence of function. Despite the extensive characterization of these cells, currently available cell surface markers allow for only a 45-fold enrichment of neural stem cells from embryonic brain. These neuronal stem cells have also been observed to generate skeletal muscle when cultured with a cell line capable of differentiating into muscle or when injected into regenerating muscle.

### Eye

The limbus is a narrow ring of tissue between the cornea and conjunctiva. Limbal stem cells give rise to the complex multilayered structure of the cornea that functions in protection, refraction and transparency **(Fig. 4.16)**. These stem cells are LRCs, form holoclones in vitro, are relatively undifferentiated, and lack CK3 and CK12 unlike the suprabasal cells of the limbus and all layers of the cornea **(Fig. 4.17)**.

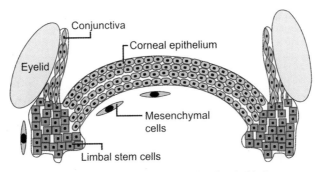

**Fig. 4.16:** In the eye, the limbal region, located between the cornea and conjunctiva is the likely stem cell zone

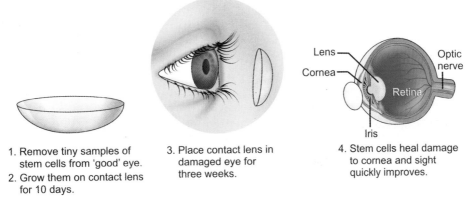

1. Remove tiny samples of stem cells from 'good' eye.
2. Grow them on contact lens for 10 days.

3. Place contact lens in damaged eye for three weeks.

4. Stem cells heal damage to cornea and sight quickly improves.

**Fig. 4.17:** Stem cell-coated contact lens restores vision to sight partially

## Heart

Anversa and Nadal-Ginard (2002) identified cells in the myocardium expressing antigens commonly found in stem cells, c-Kit, Sca-1 and MDR1. These cells were clonogenic *in vitro*, able to produce cardiomyocytes, endothelia and smooth muscle cells from single cells; they could also contribute to all these three lineages following intracardiac injection in a model of infarction. Putative stem cells have also been isolated from human heart **(Fig. 4.18)**. Very recently, Laugwitz et al (2005) have isolated what appear to be cardiac progenitors (cardioblasts) from rodent and human hearts based on the expression of the LIM-homeodomain transcription factor islet-1 (isl1). These cells decreased in frequency postnatally, but they could be expanded and differentiated *in vitro* into seemingly functional cardiomyocytes.

- Muscle stem cells, from adult muscle biopsy, can be grown out and then injected into a damaged heart, causing the heart to repair itself. This is being done in clinical trials now **(Fig. 4.19)**.

*Self-donated cells now used to repair damaged heart muscle.*

*Note*: These are still OLD cells.

## Skeletal Muscle Stem Cells

The satellite cell has been defined as a quiescent mononucleated cell ensheathed under the basal lamina that surrounds multinucleated muscle fibers **(Fig. 4.20)**. Such cells are widely thought to constitute a reserve of stem cells for muscle regeneration. Numerous studies have shown that satellite cells can be activated induced to proliferate and contribute to intact skeletal muscle fibers even after extensive tissue doublings. Moreover, these cells can be

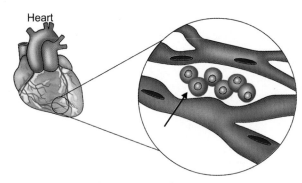

**Fig. 4.18:** Putative cardiac stem cells are found in clusters between cardiomyocytes

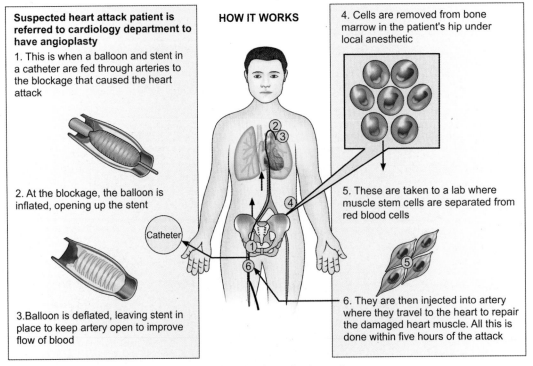

**HOW IT WORKS**

**Suspected heart attack patient is referred to cardiology department to have angioplasty**

1. This is when a balloon and stent in a catheter are fed through arteries to the blockage that caused the heart attack

2. At the blockage, the balloon is inflated, opening up the stent

3. Balloon is deflated, leaving stent in place to keep artery open to improve flow of blood

4. Cells are removed from bone marrow in the patient's hip under local anesthetic

5. These are taken to a lab where muscle stem cells are separated from red blood cells

6. They are then injected into artery where they travel to the heart to repair the damaged heart muscle. All this is done within five hours of the attack

**Fig. 4.19:** Skeletal muscle stem cells

separated from single fibers, plated in culture and induced to divide and differentiate into myotubes. The Pax7 knockout mouse apparently lacks satellite cells, but whether it is capable of regenerating muscle after damage in adulthood remains to be determined. Evidence is also accumulating the satellite cells are not alike instead are heterogeneous in the genes they express; consequently the markers of such cells are not consistent. Thus, it is clear that tissue specific stem cells exist in skeletal muscle that can contribute to muscle growth and repair, exhibit reduced proliferative capacity with increasing age of the donor, and are rapidly depleted in chronic muscle degenerative diseases such as Duchenne muscular dystrophy.

## Lung

The lung is a complex three-dimensional structure composed of a branching system of airways that serve to conduct the inspired air to the distal alveolar capillary units (air sacs). Progress in identifying lung stem cells has been impeded by the slow turnover of airway and alveolar epithelium, but the consensus view is that there is no single multipotential stem cell for the lung, but rather there are regiospecific stem cell zones in the proximal and distal lung. In the lung, a number of candidate stem cells have been proposed **(Fig. 4.21)**. In the proximal airways, scattered basal cells and cells located in the ducts of submucosal glands are likely stem cells. More proximally, pollutant-resistant Clara cells either amongst pulmonary neuroendocrine cells (*PNECs*) in neuroepithelial bodies (*NEBs*) or close to bronchoalveolar duct junctions (*BADJs*) appear to have a stem cell function. In the alveoli, proliferative type II pneumocytes replenish lost type I cells.

## Esophagus

The surface of the human esophagus is relatively flat, but invaginations of the basement membrane produce tall papillary structures within the stratified epithelium. Cell proliferation is confined to the basal and immediately epibasal layers, with cell division more common in the papillary basal layer (PBL) than in the flat interpapillary basal layer (IBL). In the PBL, the mitotic axes tend to be parallel to the basement membrane,

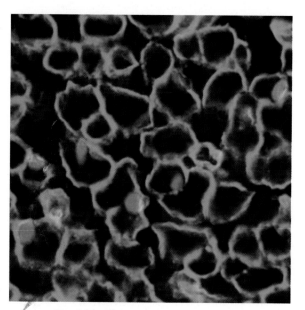

**Fig. 4.20:** Microscopic muscle stem cells

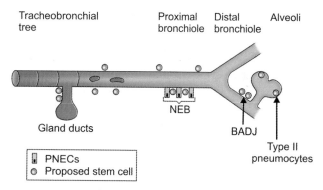

**Fig. 4.21:** Stem cells in lung

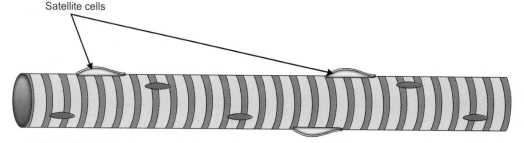

**Fig. 4.22:** Satellite cells are located between the multinucleated myotube and the cell membrane, proliferating after damage, with cell progeny becoming incorporated into the myotube

so both daughter cells remain in the basal layer, whereas in the IBL, the mitotic axes tend to be at right angles to the basement membrane; thus, one daughter cell remains a stem cell and the other daughter cell becomes a transit amplifying cell in the more proliferative active epibasal layers. Unlike the cells of the PBL and epibasal cells, esophageal stem cells are thought to be relatively undifferentiated **(Fig. 4.22)**.

## Stomach

In the stomach, the epithelial lining is folded to form structures called gastric glands; the gastric stem cells are located and maintained within a mesenchymal niche situated towards the center of the gland. Thus, cell flux in the glands is bidirectional, cells descending downwards toward the gland base and upwards toward the surface via the gastric pit.

## Intestinal Epithelium

The small intestine is composed of ciliated villi, each surrounded by crypts, embedded in the intestinal wall for protection **(Fig. 4.23)**. Each crypt is composed of about 250 simple epithelial cells that include the stem cell compartment for replenishing the villi. The multipotent stem cells are located near or at the base of each crypt. To maintain homeostasis, slow cycling stem cells are converted to rapidly but transiently proliferating cells that move to the midsegment and subsequently differentiate into either the absorptive brush-border enterocytes, mucus secreting goblet cells, or enter endocrine cells of the villi. The differentiated cells eventually die and are shed from the villi into the lumen of the gut. Crypt stem cells also produce Paneth cells at the base of the crypt, which synthesize and secrete antimicrobial peptides, digestive enzymes and growth factors. These cells are eventually cleared from the crypt by phagocytosis **(Fig. 4.24)**.

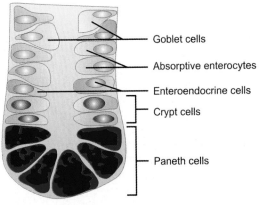

**Fig. 4.23:** Intestinal epithelium

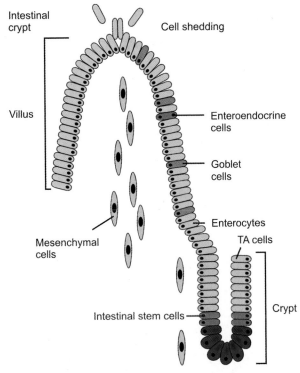

**Fig. 4.24:** Stem cells in intestine

## Pancreas

The pancreas is essentially two different tissues the exocrine pancreas, organized into acini and a branching duct system that produces digestive enzymes, and the endocrine tissue, the islets of Langerhans, that produce the hormones glucagon, insulin, somatostatin and pancreatic polypeptide from four separate cell types, $\alpha$, $\beta$, $\delta$ and PP cells, respectively **(Fig. 4.25)**. There are about 1 million islets in a human pancreas, each composed of roughly 3,000 cells of which 75% are insulin-producing $\beta$-cells. It is the renewal of $\beta$-cells that is of primary interest for the treatment of diabetes, a disease that currently afflicts 200 million people worldwide **(Fig. 4.26)**.

Seaberg et al (2004) have described clonal colonies derived with equal frequency (~2 colonies/104 cells) from both ducts and islets of mouse pancreas, and from both the nestin-positive and -negative fractions of these cell types. These cells were called pancreas-derived multipotent precursors (PMPs); clonal colonies expressed markers of the three neural lineages and all pancreatic lineages. The islets have been suggested as a location of stem cells for $\beta$-cell replacement in many species.

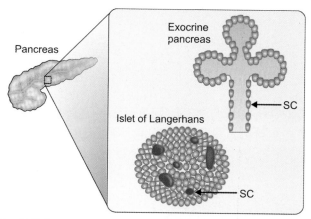

**Fig. 4.25:** Pancreas has both exocrine (ducted gland) and endocrine (islets of Langerhans) components. Both ducts and islets appear able to generate new endocrine tissue, particularly new insulin-producing β-cells

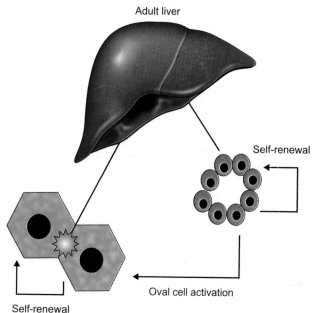

**Fig. 4.27:** In the liver, hepatocytes that make up the bulk (90%) of the liver are the regenerative cells after most injuries, but when hepatocytes regeneration is impeded some bile duct cells give rise to oval cells (TACs) that can differentiate into hepatocytes

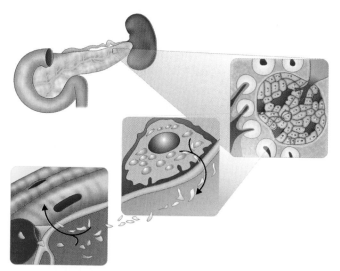

**Fig. 4.26:** Insulin production in the human pancreas

# Hepatic Stem Cells

Despite the fact that the liver is an organ capable of extensive regeneration, the precise source of the tissue specific stem cells responsible for this regeneration remains unclear. In contrast to bone marrow or skin in which a relatively small population of cells undergoes massive expansion to support regeneration, liver regeneration following partial hepatectomy, in which two-thirds of the liver of a rat is removed, involves a modest proliferation by a variety of differentiated liver cells including hepatocytes, biliary epithelial cells, and endothelial cells **(Fig. 4.27)**. However, following some types of injury which compromise hepatocytes, a smaller portion of stem-like

cells near the bile ducts give rise to a proliferation of oval cells that subsequently generate hepatocytes and ductular cells. These data, taken together with morphological studies of liver regeneration following injury, have raised the possibility that the true liver stem cell with multilineage potential resides in or near the terminal bile ductules.

## Kidney

The kidney has a low rate of cell turnover under steady state conditions, but can regenerate tubular epithelium after injury. The identity of any renal stem cells has not been readily forthcoming. Since the kidney develops centrifugally, the medulla is the oldest region and thus could be the location of a stem cell niche. These cells were capable of *in vitro* expansion and differentiation into epithelia and endothelia, and formed tubular structures and endothelia in the damaged kidneys of SCID mice.

## Mammary Glands

As in many tissues, the identity of stem cells in the mammalian breast is the subject of controversy. The collective wisdom is that they reside in the terminal ductal lobulo-alveolar units (TDLUs) as small undifferentiated cells in the luminal cell layer that do not make contact with the lumen. These cells are bipotential, giving rise to luminal and myoepithelial cells (**Figs 4.28 and 4.29**).

### Cervix

Surprisingly little is known about the identity of the stem cells proposed to maintain the lining of the female genital tract such as that of the vagina and uterus. The uterus is lined principally by the endometrium, an epithelial lining thrown into deep fold s that vary in depth dependent on the menstrual cycle. This gives way to the endocervical canal of the uterine cervix, lined by a simple columnar epithelium, again with contiguous glands: the endocervical crypts. At the neck of the uterus, the simple columnar epithelium gives way, at the so-called transformation zone, to the stratified squamous epithelium of the ectocervix. The acidic vaginal environment results in squamous metaplasia of the transformation zone, preceded by the appearance of sub-columnar reserve cells that undergo hyperplasia before forming metaplastic squamous epithelium indistinguishable from the squamous epithelia of the ectocervix. Like the basal cells of the original squamous epithelium, these reserve cells have round nuclei and little cytoplasm.

### Testis

In the mammalian testis, the mitotic divisions occur amongst the various generations of so-called type A spermatogonia that are located on the basement membrane of the seminiferous tubule the meiotic reduction divisions and further differentiation towards terminally differentiated

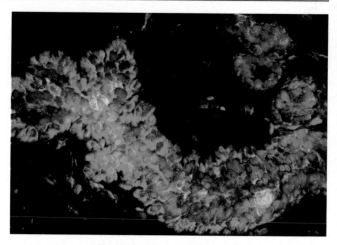

**Fig. 4.29:** Mammary stem cells

spermatozoa occurs centripetally (**Fig. 4.30**). Spermatogonia that are relatively devoid of heterochromatin are called Apale, and those occurring as single cells (incidence of ~2 in 104 testicular cells) are probably the stem cells. Their distribution is not random in mouse and rat; rather they are located in those areas of seminiferous tubules that border on interstitial tissue (**Figs 4.31 and 4.32**).

### Prostate

Anatomically the prostate gland varies greatly between species, but can essentially be described as an exocrine gland enveloping the urethra at the base of the bladder, composed of blind-ending tubules that open into the urethra. In the mouse, based on the location of LRCs, prostatic

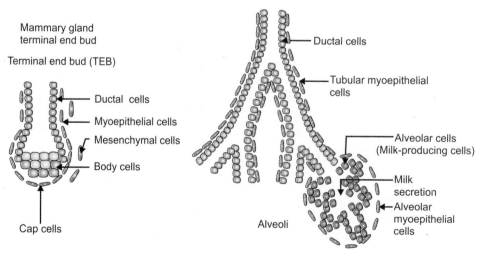

**Fig. 4.28:** Stem cells are thought to be located in the terminal ductule lobuloalveolar units (TDLUs, *boxed area*) as small cells that do not make contact with the luminal surface

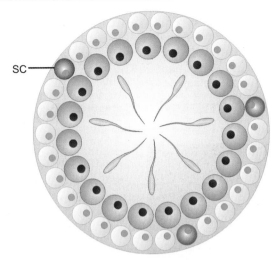

**Fig. 4.30:** In the seminiferous epithelium, stem cells and TACs all reside on the basement membrane as various generations of spermatogonia

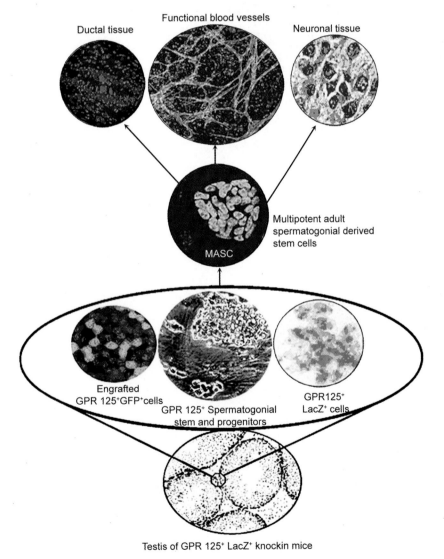

**Fig. 4.31:** Generation of organ-specific tissues from GPR 125 + multipotent adult spermatogonital-derived stem cells (MASCs)

epithelial stem cells are thought to be in the proximal regions of prostatic ducts, close to the urethra. Human prostatic stem cells are thought to be multipotential, able to generate secretory, basal and neuroendocrine cells, located amongst basal cells that form a continuous layer between the luminal secretory cells and the basement membrane.

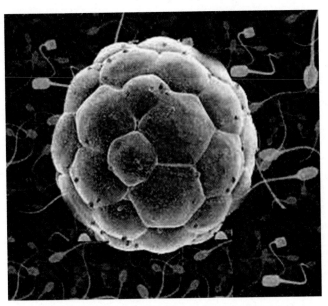

**Fig. 4.32:** Sperms could be the next stem cells source

## Skin

Both the epidermis and hair follicle require stem cells to support high rates of epithelial turnover. Several epidermal injuries revealed that keratinocytes can migrate from the hair follicles to regenerate the epidermis. Furthermore, several recent papers contend that keratinocytes stem cells that give rise to both epidermis and hair follicles reside in a specific region of the follicular epithelium, the bulge zone, where they cycle slowly, express keratin K5 and K14, and generate progeny to replenish the epidermal basal layer **(Figs 4.33 and 4.34)**.

## LIMITATIONS OF ADULT STEM CELL THERAPY

1. Human adult stem cells are rare and it is difficult to isolate a unique group of stem cells in pure form. So it is not surprising that what at first appears to be plasticity in a single adult stem cell type could be the result of a mixture of cells of different types, including different types of stem cells.
2. The environment in which stem cells grow or are placed to grow has an important but poorly understood effect on their fate—a theme that was echoed by many speakers at the workshop.
3. The relationship of the cellular environment to the concept of plasticity in adult stem cells.

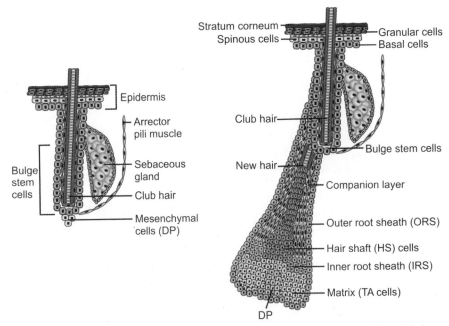

**Fig. 4.33:** In the epidermis, stem cells are present in the interfollicular epidermis (*IFE*) and bulge region

Researchers have developed a technique for creating stem cells without the controversial use of eggs or embryos

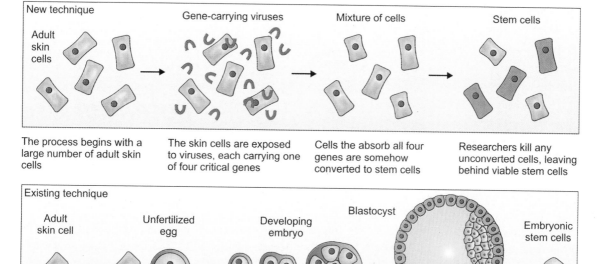

**New technique**

Adult skin cells · Gene-carrying viruses · Mixture of cells · Stem cells

The process begins with a large number of adult skin cells

The skin cells are exposed to viruses, each carrying one of four critical genes

Cells the absorb all four genes are somehow converted to stem cells

Researchers kill any unconverted cells, leaving behind viable stem cells

**Existing technique**

Adult skin cell · Unfertilized egg · Developing embryo · Blastocyst · Embryonic stem cells

Inner cell mass

In the therapeutic cloning, the nucleus of an adult skin cell is inserted into an unfertilized egg with its nucleus removed

The egg reprograms the adult nucleus back to its embryonic state and the egg begins to divide

After several days a blastocyst forms. Stem cells can be taken from the blastocyst's inner cell mass, which destroys the embryo

**Fig. 4.34:** From skin cells to stem cells

4. Most studies inadequately demonstrate that stem cells have produced a functionally useful cell in the organ. Most studies showing the plasticity of stem cells rely on the detection of proteins in the newly generated tissues that are commonly associated with a particular type of differentiated cell. But there is no consensus in the scientific community that the detection of a particular protein constitutes sufficient evidence that the cells and tissues formed are, in fact, fully functional and normal.

5. Inability to maintain these cells in culture for very long before they differentiate into their mature progeny. One can envision two therapeutic approaches to stem cells. In the first, stem cells themselves are implanted in a diseased or injured organ in the hope that they will give rise to the mature cells needed by that organ. In the second, the stem cells are stimulated to differentiate into the needed mature tissue outside the body, and that tissue is implanted in the organ. Those adult stem cells are difficult to isolate, purify, and culture causes problems for either approach, although even the ability to culture stem cells for a limited time, including in the presence of other cells, could have therapeutic potential.

6. Finally, the implications of what is known about *human adult* stem cells are often overlooked amid reports of successes with experiments in rodents that simulate heart attack, retinal disease, and diabetes. Confirmed reports of truly multipotent human adult stem cells are scarce. Without conclusive identification, the existence of a multipotent fat cell remains unconfirmed.

# CHAPTER 5

# *Potential Uses of Human Stem Cells*

There are many ways in which human stem cells can be used in basic research and in clinical research. However, there are many technical hurdles between the promise of stem cells and the realization of these uses, which will only be overcome by continued intensive stem cell research.

Studies of human embryonic stem cells may yield information about the complex events that occur during human development. A primary goal of this work is to identify how undifferentiated stem cells become differentiated. Scientists know that turning genes on and off is central to this process. Some of the most serious medical conditions, such as cancer and birth defects, are due to abnormal cell division and differentiation. A better understanding of the genetic and molecular controls of these processes may yield information about how such diseases arise and suggest new strategies for therapy. A significant hurdle to this use and most uses of stem cells is that scientists do not yet fully understand the signals that turn specific genes on and off to influence the differentiation of the stem cell **(Figs 5.1 and 5.2)**.

## CURRENT TREATMENTS

Different regulatory frameworks apply depending on the mode of action of the treatment. A distinction is made between those treatments where the stem cells produce a therapeutic substance resulting in a medicinal action and

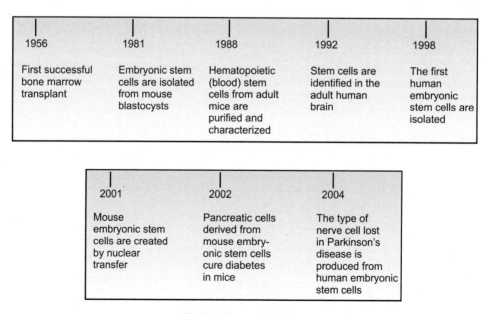

**Fig. 5.1:** Stem cell timeline

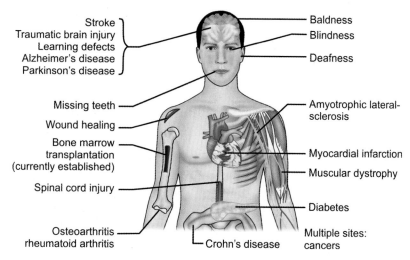

**Fig. 5.2:** Potential uses of stem cells

those (nonmedicinal) treatments where stem cells replace or augment normal tissue function. Current treatment options for such diseases include:

- *Long-term drug therapy*: Human stem cells could also be used to test new drugs. For example, new medications could be tested for safety on differentiated cells generated from human pluripotent cell lines. Other kinds of cell lines are already used in this way. Cancer cell lines, for example, are used to screen potential antitumor drugs. But, the availability of pluripotent stem cells would allow drug testing in a wider range of cell types. However, to screen drugs effectively, the conditions must be identical when comparing different drugs. Therefore, scientists will have to be able to precisely control the differentiation of stem cells into the specific cell type on which drugs will be tested. Current knowledge of the signals controlling differentiation fall well short of being able to mimic these conditions precisely to consistently have identical differentiated cells for each drug being tested. New studies indicate that it may be possible to direct the differentiation of human embryonic stem cells in cell culture to form insulin-producing cells that eventually could be used in transplantation therapy for diabetics.
- *Transplants*: Perhaps the most important potential application of human stem cells is the generation of cells and tissues that could be used for cell-based therapies. Today, donated organs and tissues are often used to replace ailing or destroyed tissue, but the need for transplantable tissues and organs far outweighs the available supply. Stem cells, directed to differentiate into specific cell types, offer the possibility of a renewable source of replacement cells and tissues to treat diseases including Parkinson's and Alzheimer's diseases, spinal cord injury, stroke, burns, heart disease, diabetes, osteoarthritis, and rheumatoid arthritis.

To realize the promise of novel cell-based therapies for such pervasive and debilitating diseases, scientists must be able to easily and reproducibly manipulate stem cells so that they possess the necessary characteristics for successful differentiation, transplantation and engraftment. The following is a list of steps in successful cell-based treatments that scientists will have to learn to precisely control to bring such treatments to the clinic. To be useful for transplant purposes, stem cells must be reproducibly made to:

- Proliferate extensively and generate sufficient quantities of tissue
- Differentiate into the desired cell type(s)
- Survive in the recipient after transplant
- Integrate into the surrounding tissue after transplant
- Function appropriately for the duration of the recipient's life
- Avoid harming the recipient in any way.

Also, to avoid the problem of immune rejection, scientists are experimenting with different research strategies to generate tissues that will not be rejected.

- Medical devices such as pacemakers, vascular grafts, orthopedic pins and prosthetic heart valves. Such devices may need replacing over the patient's lifetime **(Fig. 5.3)**.

## Parkinson's Disease

It is the second most common neurodegenerative disorder and affects almost 1 percent of the population above the

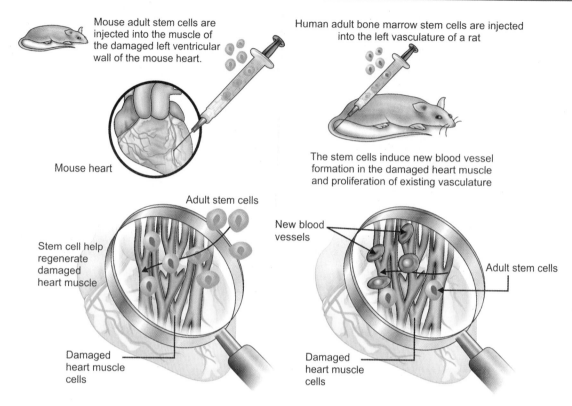

**Fig. 5.3:** Heart muscle repair with adult stem cells

age of 60. Patients primarily suffer from motor symptoms such as bradykinesia (slowness of movement), rigidity (muscle stiffness) and tremor at rest. These symptoms progress over time and, in addition, most patients eventually exhibit vegetative disturbances, depression and dementia in the course of the disease. The main neuropathological finding in PD is the progressive loss of dopaminergic (DA) neurons in the substantia nigra pars compacta (SNc). These neurons project to the striatum and their loss results in a reduction of striatal dopamine (DA) levels **(Fig. 5.4)**.

Stem cells offer hope to those with Parkinson's disease, which is caused by the loss of nerve cells in the brain. These nerve cells produce a neurotransmitter called dopamine. If stem cells can be cultivated to become these dopamine-producing nerve cells, researchers believe that they could replace the lost cells. In this disease the human embryonic VM is dissected from embryos from routine abortions after informed consent of the woman undergoing abortion and according to ethical guidelines. The tissue is enzymatically and mechanically dissociated in some centers, in others the tissue is stored for several weeks and implanted as tissue strands, or the tissue is grafted in pieces. The cells are stereotactically injected into the putamen and caudate.

Patients have been grafted uni- and bilaterally. Immuno-suppression of the patient varies between centers. The cells are injected along several trajectories. Tissue from two to four embryos/side of the brain is needed to achieve a sufficient number of surviving DA neurons **(Fig. 5.5)**.

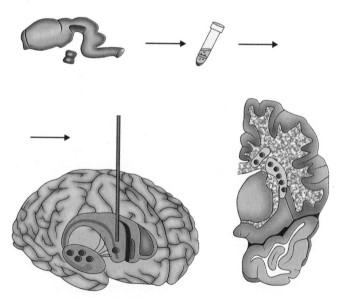

**Fig. 5.4:** Stem cells in Parkinson's disease

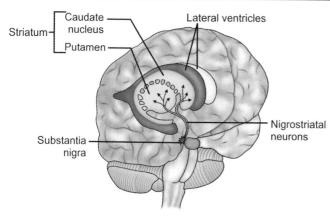

**Fig. 5.5:** Parkinson's disease

## Diabetes Mellitus

The pathology of type 1 diabetes is caused by the auto-immune destruction or malfunction of pancreatic $\beta$ cells, and consequently, a lack of insulin. The absence of insulin is life-threatening, thus requiring diabetic patients to take daily hormone injections from exogenous sources; however, insulin injections do not adequately mimic $\beta$ cell function. This results in the development of diabetic complications such as neuropathy, nephropathy, retinopathy and diverse cardiovascular disorders. New studies indicate that it may be possible to direct the differentiation of human embryonic stem cells in cell culture to form insulin-producing cells that eventually could be used in transplantation therapy for diabetics.

The field of generating new $\beta$-cells from stem cells, either embryonic or adult, is still in its infancy. Each new report has been met with a mixture of excitement and scepticism. With continued efforts and rigorous assessments, hopefully the potential of generating enough new cells from stem cells will be realized **(Fig. 5.6)**.

## NONMEDICINAL THERAPIES

Most current stem cell therapies are nonmedicinal in nature, and act principally by replacing, repairing or regenerating some function of the patient's body.

- *Unmodified stem cells used in transplants*: The simplest therapies involve transplanting tissue containing stem cells into a patient. Examples include bone marrow transplants, placental stem cells (which have been used in the US to treat a variety of diseases) and fetal stem cells (used to treat Parkinson's disease with limited success).
- Stem cells that have been extensively manipulated/ modified or subject to an engineering process: Such cells

can be used to replace (bones, heart valves, blood vessels and arteries), repair (neurological tissue, skin, or muscle) or regenerate (liver and pancreas) human tissue.

## STEM CELL RESEARCH AND REGENERATIVE MEDICINE

### Introduction

Stem cells have recently been heralded by the media as a promising new tool in the fight of degenerative diseases. However, much knowledge stands to be gained before stem cell therapies can be used as commonplace. A full understanding of stem cells in their many forms and the progeny they give rise to are paramount to their future use. Much attention has been paid to human embryonic stem cells (hESCs). Since the initial discovery of hESCs, other stem cell sources have been discovered one of which is hEGCs, these cells are a possible substitute with shown pluripotent ability. Human embryonic germ cells can also serve as an additional tool for fighting disease.

### Primordial Germ Cells

Embryonic germ cells (EGCs) are the derivatives of primordial germs cells (PGCs). They are isolated from the gonadal ridge and mesenchyma of fetal tissue. PGCs are the embryonic precursors of gametes and when allowed to mature they will form the sperm and egg cells. PGCs are first identifiable at the base of the allantois in the 7-day mouse embryo as a cluster of approximately eight cells. From there, the PGCs invade the endoderm, migrate through the hindgut and ultimately settle into the genital ridge. Migration within the hindgut requires the Stem Cell Factor (SCF)/c-kit inter-action. Migration out of the hindgut and into the genital ridge occurs during day 9.5 of the developing mouse embryo and it appears to be directed by factors produced by the genital ridge **(Figs 5.7 and 5.8)**. One such factor which is important in attracting PGCs to the genital ridge is the peptide growth factor Stromal Derived Factor 1 (SDF-1), which is produced by the stromal cells of the genital ridge and gonads and which interacts with the receptor CXCR4 receptor expressed on PGCs.

### EGC and ESC Properties

Embryonic germ cells (EGCs) and embryonic stem cells (ESCs) have several similar characteristics. Both cell types replicate for an extended period of time, show no chromosomal abnormalities and express a set of markers regarded as characteristic of pluripotent cells. When culture condi-

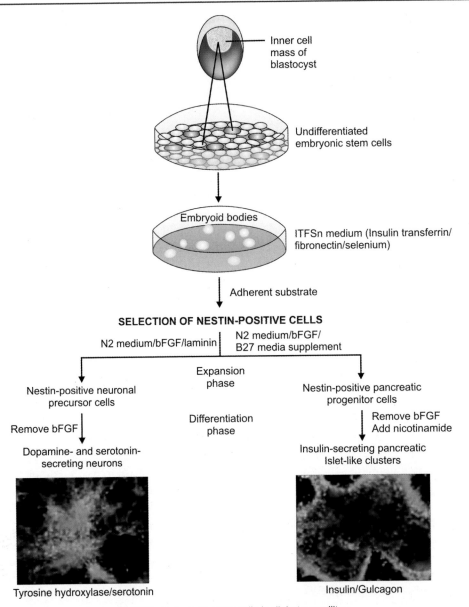

Inner cell mass of blastocyst

Undifferentiated embryonic stem cells

Embryoid bodies

ITFSn medium (Insulin transferrin/ fibronectin/selenium)

Adherent substrate

**SELECTION OF NESTIN-POSITIVE CELLS**

N2 medium/bFGF/laminin

N2 medium/bFGF/ B27 media supplement

Nestin-positive neuronal precursor cells

Expansion phase

Nestin-positive pancreatic progenitor cells

Remove bFGF

Differentiation phase

Remove bFGF Add nicotinamide

Dopamine- and serotonin- secreting neurons

Insulin-secreting pancreatic Islet-like clusters

Tyrosine hydroxylase/serotonin

Insulin/Gulcagon

**Fig. 5.6:** Embryonic stem cells in diabetes mellitus

tions are adjusted to allow differentiation, both EGC and ESC cells can spontaneously differentiate into derivatives of the primary germ layers, endoderm, mesoderm and ectoderm. In contrast, the ESCs are derived from the inner cell mass of a 5-day old embryo whereas EGCs are derived from the gonadal ridge of the 5-9 week foetus. Additional experiments using hESCs have shown the formation of teratomas. This illustration of teratoma formation is used as standard evidence of hESC pluripotency when injected into an NOD/SCID (immunosuppressed) mouse. While hESC are known to produce teratomas, the engraftment of hEGCs into immunosuppressed mice will not actually generate teratomas. In fact, embryonic stem cells and embryonic germ cells from select species have been shown to form teratomas when injected. Conversely hEGCs have yet to display this behavior. To date, teratomas from analysis of *in vivo* hEGCs have not yet been observed.

## Imprinting

The imprinting status of EGCs is a major issue of concern in their potential for clinical use. Imprinting is the epigenetic change of DNA in which expression of only one of the parental alleles is evident. Epigenetic changes, which are the alteration of proteins surrounding DNA but not the DNA itself, involve

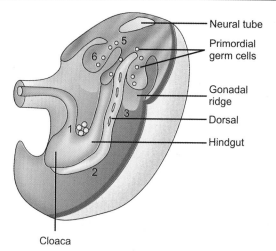

**Fig. 5.7:** Transverse section of embryo showing the migratory path of PGCs from cloaca (1), past the dorsal (6) and up toward the neural tube (5)

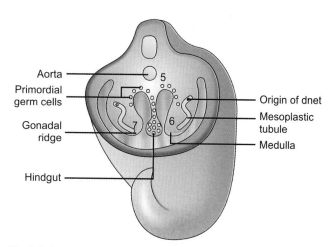

**Fig. 5.8:** Longitudinal section of embryo showing the latter part of the migratory path of PGCs from the hindgut up toward the aorta (5) and down into gonadal ridge (7)

DNA methylation and histone modification. Imprinting is necessary for normal function and involves about 100 imprinting genes. Erasure of the imprints is necessary between generations so that gametes of both sexes can be formed and expressed. Also it is important so that proper expression can occur when two sets of DNA combine. Studies with mouse EGCs show that tissues or differentiated cells from EGCs frequently do not exhibit imprinting genes properly. Studies with human EGCs appear altered, and more importantly show normal imprinting. Understanding when erasure occurs is essential to harvesting EGCs without imprinting erasure for therapeutic use **(Fig. 5.9)**. It is believed that erasure can start as early as during movement towards the genital ridge. However, most of the demethylation of PGCs occurs within one day of entering the gonadal ridge.

## Human EGC Derivation

To understand how human EGCs were developed, it is important to recognize preliminary EGC work done in mice. Murine EGCs were derived years before human EGCs were, and it was the culturing conditions and characterization techniques developed for murine cells that were the basis for human EGC derivation **(Fig. 5.10)**. Important factors like stem cell factor (SCF), (LIF), and (bFGF) were found to enhance murine primordial germ cell (PGC) replication and survival, making them key for culturing. The PGC culture formed colonies of cells resembling murine ESCs. Initial characterization showed that cells were positive for markers such as SSEA-1. The cells could also be maintained on feeder layers.

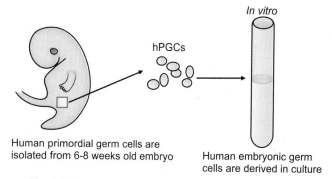

Human primordial germ cells are isolated from 6-8 weeks old embryo

Human embryonic germ cells are derived in culture

**Fig. 5.9:** Embryonic germ cell derivation from 6 to 8 weeks old embryo for experimental investigations

Human EGCs were first derived in 1998 by a group led by John Gearhart. The gonadal ridges and mesenteries of 5 to 9 weeks fetuses, from therapeutically terminated pregnancies, were mechanically and chemically disaggregated, passaged on mouse fibroblast feeder cells and then cultured in growth medium containing fetal bovine serum (FBS), LIF, bFGF, and forskolin. A significant portion of the cells were positive for AP, had markers similar of ESCs (SSEA-1, SSEA-3, SSEA-4, TRA-1-60, and TRA-1-81), and were morphologically similar to murine EGCs. The cells were also shown to have normal and stable karyotype for over 10 passages. When culturing the embryoid bodies (EB) without LIF, bFGF and forskolin, the pluripotency of the cells became apparent *in vitro*. The result was a growth of a variety of cells from each germ layer, accordingly meeting important criteria for pluripotency. Later, other groups also derived human EGCs using similar methods. The EGCs

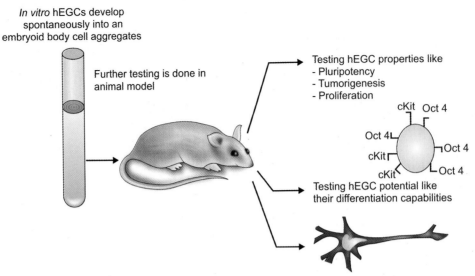

*In vitro* hEGCs develop spontaneously into an embryoid body cell aggregates

Further testing is done in animal model

Testing hEGC properties like
- Pluripotency
- Tumorigenesis
- Proliferation

Testing hEGC potential like their differentiation capabilities

**Fig. 5.10:** Collected hEGCs are grafted into mice to test properties, e.g. pluripotency, tumorigenesis, proliferation and differentiation potential

were further characterized to show Oct-4 expression and telomerase activity, both of which are both important ESC properties.

## Proliferation

PGCs can be transiently cultured on feeder cell layers expressing the transmembrane-bound isoform of SCF. SCF, together with LIF, promote PGC survival by suppressing apoptosis. Basic fibroblast growth factor (bFGF) is also active in PGC cultures, promoting germ cell proliferation. If PGCs are cultured with SLF, LIF, and bFGF, they can form cell lines termed EGCs. This could be attributed to the fact that hEGCs have been less successful at generating long-term, robust cultures as described earlier. It has been shown that they do not have quite the same set of pluripotency, or "stemness" markers as hESCs, which suggests they may be more mature or slightly more differentiated than hESCs **(Fig. 5.11)**. The loss of stemness as EGCs remain in culture may be due to EGCs continuing to follow PGC fate in the embryo or imprinting alteration and erasure in culture.

## Clinical Applications

Human EGCs spontaneously form EBs in culture as testament to their pluripotent capabilities. Embryonic Body cells (EBCs) are clusters of cells formed when the EGCs aggregate and randomly differentiate into precursors of the embryonic germ cell layers, simulating an environment of early embryonic development. Unfortunately, the only definitive way to ascertain a stem cell's pluripotency is from the formation of chimeric offspring (in trials with mice), but due to ethical considerations this is not practical with hEGC lines. The goal of current research is to develop "normal" cells that have the ability to function *in vivo*. EB formation is essential for applications in regenerative medicine, because it is a stepping stone towards the derivation of other cell lineages. *In vitro* experiments with EGC-derived EBCs have been promising in yielding neuronal and musculoskeletal cells. In neuronal differentiation, EGC-derived EBCs in culture were shown to express typical neuronal progenitor markers such as nestin and N-CAM, while "stem" indicative markers such as Oct-4 and hTERT were undetectable. When prolonged in culture, the cells began to physically resemble neurons, generating long tubular projections to interconnect with other cell aggregates. In another study their gene expression and protein synthesis were shown to follow chondrogenic and mesenchymal differentiation patterns.

Of particular clinical interest are hEGC *in vivo* experiments, which are limited in number. Recently, hEGC derived EBCs cultured for neuronal differentiation were implanted into damaged neural tissue in paralyzed rats. Over a period of time, the transplanted animals regained function whereas the controls remained paralyzed. This could not be directly attributed to the function of the implanted cells, although they are thought to have directed regrowth and prevented neural cell death. More recently, hEGC-derived

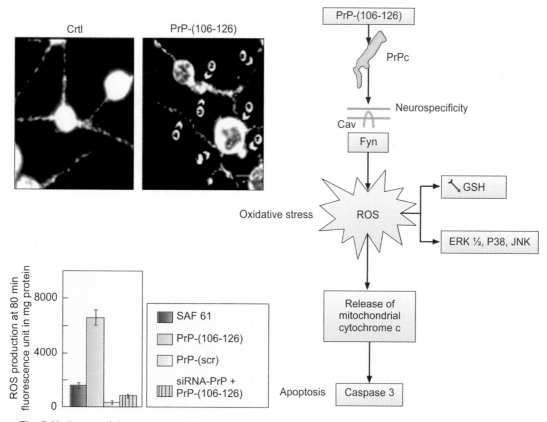

**Fig. 5.11:** Impact of the neurotoxic PrP-(106-126) peptide on the intracellular targets of PrP$^c$ in neuronal cells

human neural stem cells (NSCs) were shown to repair brain damage in newborn mice. This suggests that the NSCs were able to engraft and repair the lost neurons. In addition, experiments have indicated that, by seeding a graft structure with hEGC derived cells, the bladder of a rat was reformed without loss of function or more importantly evidence of graft rejection.

These preliminary studies with human embryonic germ cells have yielded very promising results for clinical application starting from nerve regeneration and beyond. hEGCs are particularly appealing because of one of their primary shortcomings, namely that they do not form teratomas upon injection. This may very well show that they are further along the differentiation pathway than embryonic stem cells (ESCs). This could be a blessing in disguise, making them much more conducive to predictable behavior *in vivo*, and thereby making hEGCs more appealing for clinical trials. Hopeful thinking aside, much research yet needs to be done before regenerative medicine with stem cells of any kind moves to a patient's bedside. Much is to be learned and characterized about the differentiation of embryonic germ cells to make them of medicinal value, and

in the process, researchers may stand to gain a greater depth of knowledge in the events of early development.

## Oocyte Renewal

The widely held dogma of female reproductive biology is that females of most mammalian species lose the ability to replenish their oocyte population altogether during fetal development. Thus, unlike their male-counterparts, females are born with a finite number of oocytes, which will be eventually become exhausted and lead to menopause. However, contrary to this long-standing belief, it has been recently shown that oogenesis, the production of new oocytes, continues into adult life. It has been demonstrated that germline stem cells (GSCs) in female mice are capable of replenishing the oocyte population in mature females. Furthermore, and even more surprisingly, it has been suggested that these GSCs in adult female mammals may actually reside in the bone marrow and peripheral blood. However, it is important to note that further research is needed to determine whether or not the putative oocytes generated from GSCs are competent for fertilization, capable of embryonic development or creation of a viable fetus.

# Stem Cells and Tissue Engineering

## TISSUE ENGINEERING

The chronic shortage of donor organs and tissues for transplantation has provided the impetus for intense research in the field of tissue engineering. Tissue engineering is the use of a combination of cells, engineering materials, and suitable biochemical factors to improve or replace biological functions.

## Definition

- Probably the first definition of tissue engineering was by Langer and Vacanti who stated it to be "An interdisciplinary field that applies the principles of engineering and life sciences toward the development of biological substitutes that restore, maintain, or improve tissue function or a whole organ".
- MacArthur and Oreffo defined tissue engineering as "Understanding the principles of tissue growth, and applying this to produce functional replacement tissue for clinical use".
- A further description goes on to say that an "Underlying supposition of tissue engineering is that the employment of natural biology of the system will allow for greater success in developing therapeutic strategies aimed at the replacement, repair, maintenance, and/or enhancement of tissue function".

While the semi-official definition of tissue engineering covers a broad range of applications, in practice the term has come to represent applications that repair or replace structural tissues (i.e. bone, cartilage, blood vessels, bladder, etc.). These are tissues that function by virtue of their mechanical properties. A closely related (and older) field is cell transplantation. This field is concerned with the transplantation of cells that perform a specific biochemical function (e.g. an artificial pancreas, or an artificial liver).

The term regenerative medicine is often used synonymously with *tissue engineering*, although those involved in regenerative medicine place more emphasis on the use of stem cells to produce tissues.

Tissue engineering solves problems by using living cells as engineering materials. These could be artificial skin that includes living fibroblasts, cartilage repaired with living chondrocytes, or other types of cells used in other ways **(Figs 6.1A and B)**. Cells became available as engineering materials when scientists at Geron Corp discovered how to extend telomeres in 1998, producing an immortalized cell line. Before this, laboratory cultures of healthy, noncancerous mammalian cells would only divide a fixed number of times, up to the Hayflick limit. From fluid tissues such as blood, cells are extracted by bulk methods, usually centrifugation or apheresis. From solid tissues, extraction is more difficult. Usually the tissue is minced, and then digested with the enzymes trypsin or collagenase to remove the extracellular matrix that holds the cells. After that, the cells are free floating, and extracted using centrifugation or aspheresis. Digestion with trypsin is very dependent on temperature. Higher temperatures digest the matrix faster, but create more damage. Collagenase is less temperature dependent, and damages fewer cells, but takes longer and is a more expensive reagent.

## CELLS USED FOR TISSUE ENGINEERING

Cells are often categorized by their source:
- *Autologous* cells are obtained from the same individual to whom they will be reimplanted. Autologous cells have the fewest problems with rejection and pathogen transmission, however, in some cases might not be available. For example, in genetic disease suitable autologous cells are not available. Also very ill or elderly

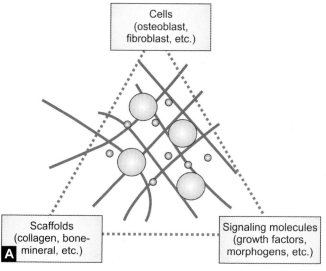
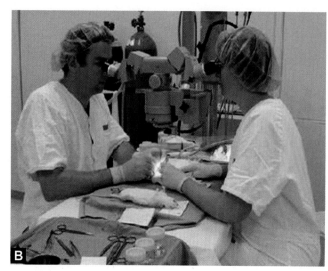

**Figs 6.1A and B:** Tissue engineering

persons, as well as patients suffering from severe burns, may not have sufficient quantities of autologous cells to establish useful cell lines. Moreover since this category of cells needs to be harvested from the patient, there are also some concerns related to the necessity of performing such surgical operations that might lead to donor site infection or chronic pain.

Autologous cells also must be cultured from samples before they can be used: this takes time, so autologous solutions may not be very quick. Recently there has been a trend towards the use of mesenchymal stem cells from bone marrow and fat. These cells can differentiate into a variety of tissue types, including bone, cartilage, fat, and nerve. A large number of cells can be easily and quickly isolated from fat, thus opening the potential for large numbers of cells to be quickly and easily obtained. Several companies have been founded to capitalize on this technology, the most successful at this time being Cytori therapeutics.

- *Allogenic* cells come from the body of a donor of the same species. While there are some ethical constraints to the use of human cells for *in vitro* studies, the employment of dermal fibroblasts from human foreskin has been demonstrated to be immunologically safe and thus a viable choice for tissue engineering of skin.
- *Xenogenic* cells are those isolated from individuals of another species. In particular animal cells have been used quite extensively in experiments aimed at the construction of cardiovascular implants.

- Syngenic' *or isogenic* cells are isolated from genetically identical organisms, such as twins, clones, or highly inbred research animal models.
- *Primary* cells are from an organism.
- *Secondary* cells are from a cell bank.
- *Stem cells* are undifferentiated cells with the ability to divide in culture and give rise to different forms of specialized cells. According to their source stem cells are divided into "adult" and "embryonic" stem cells, the first class being multipotent and the latter mostly pluripotent; some cells are totipotent, in the earliest stages of the embryo. While there is still a large ethical debate related with the use of embryonic stem cells, it is thought that stem cells may be useful for the repair of diseased or damaged tissues, or may be used to grow new organs **(Fig. 6.2)**.

## ENGINEERING MATERIALS

Cells as found above are generally implanted or "seeded" into an artificial structure capable of supporting three-dimensional tissue formation. These scaffolds are often critical, both *ex vivo* as well as *in vivo*, to recapitulating the *in vivo* milieu and allowing cells to influence their own microenvironments. Such devices, usually referred to as **scaffolds**, serve at least one of the following purposes:
- Allow cell attachment and migration
- Deliver and retain cells and biochemical factors
- Enable diffusion of vital cell nutrients and expressed products

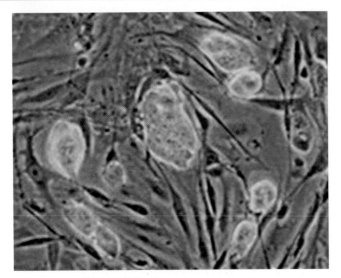

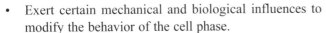

Fig. 6.2: Mouse embryonic stem cells

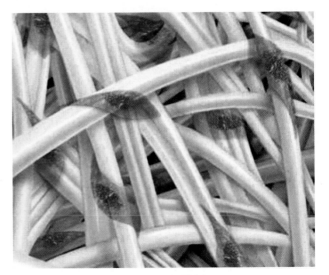

Fig. 6.3: Scaffolds

- Exert certain mechanical and biological influences to modify the behavior of the cell phase.

To achieve the goal of tissue reconstruction, scaffolds must meet some specific requirements. A high porosity and an adequate pore size are necessary to facilitate cell seeding and diffusion throughout the whole structure of both cells and nutrients. Biodegradability is essential since scaffolds need to be absorbed by the surrounding tissues without the necessity of a surgical removal. The rate at which degradation occurs has to coincide as much as possible with the rate of tissue formation: this means that while cells are fabricating their own natural matrix structure around themselves, the scaffold is able to provide structural integrity within the body and eventually it will breakdown leaving the neotissue, newly formed tissue which will takeover the mechanical load. Injectability is also important for clinical uses.

Many different materials (natural and synthetic, biodegradable and permanent) have been investigated. Most of these materials have been known in the medical field before the advent of tissue engineering as a research topic, being already employed as bioresorbable sutures. Examples of these materials are collagen or some linear aliphatic polyester.

New biomaterials have been engineered to have ideal properties and functional customization: injectability, synthetic manufacture, biocompatibility, non-immunogenicity, transparency, nanoscale fibers, low concentration, resorption rates, etc.

- PuraMatrix, originating from the MIT labs of Zhang, Rich, Grodzinsky and Langer is one of these new biomimetic scaffold families which has now been commercialized and is impacting clinical tissue engineering.
- A commonly used synthetic material is PLA—polylactic acid. This is polyester which degrades within the human body to form lactic acid, a naturally occurring chemical which is easily removed from the body.
- Similar materials are polyglycolic acid (PGA) and polycaprolactone (PCL): their degradation mechanism is similar to that of PLA, but they exhibit respectively a faster and a slower rate of degradation compared to PLA.

Scaffolds may also be constructed from natural materials **(Fig. 6.3)**: in particular different derivatives of the extracellular matrix have been studied to evaluate their ability to support cell growth. Protein materials, such as collagen or fibrin, and polysaccharide materials, like chitosan or glycosaminoglycans (GAGs), have all proved suitable in terms of cell compatibility, but some issues with potential immunogenicity still remains. Among GAGs hyaluronic acid, possibly in combination with cross-linking agents (e.g. glutaraldehyde, water soluble carbodiimide, etc.), is one of the possible choices as scaffold material. Functionalized groups of scaffolds may be useful in the delivery of small molecules (drugs) to specific tissues **(Figs 6.4 and 6.5)**.

## SYNTHESIS OF TISSUE ENGINEERING SCAFFOLDS

A number of different methods have been described in literature for preparing porous structures to be employed

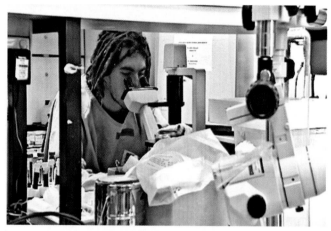

**Fig. 6.4:** Stem cells used for tissue engineering

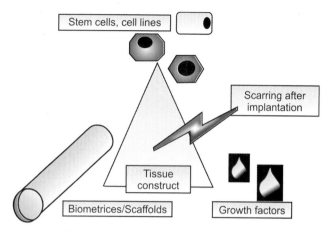

**Fig. 6.6:** Helpful triplet in tissue engineering

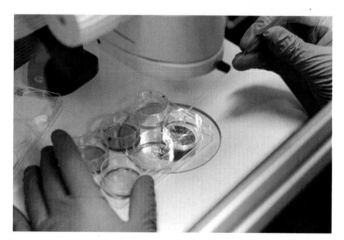

**Fig. 6.5:** Isolation of cells

as tissue engineering scaffolds **(Fig. 6.6)**. Each of these techniques presents its own advantages, but none is devoid of drawbacks.

- *Nanofiber self-assembly*: Molecular self-assembly is one of the few methods to create biomaterials with properties similar in scale and chemistry to that of the natural *in vivo* extracellular matrix (ECM). Moreover, these hydrogel scaffolds have shown superior *in vivo* toxicology and biocompatibility compared with traditional macroscaffolds and animal-derived materials. PuraMatrix synthetic peptide hydrogels exemplify this category.

- *Textile technologies*: These techniques include all the approaches that have been successfully employed for the preparation of non-woven meshes of different polymers. In particular non-woven polyglycolide structures have been tested for tissue engineering applications: such fibrous structures have been found

useful to grow different types of cells. The principal drawbacks are related to the difficulties of obtaining high porosity and regular pore size.

- *Solvent casting and particulate leaching (SCPL)*: This approach allows the preparation of porous structures with regular porosity, but with a limited thickness. First the polymer is dissolved into a suitable organic solvent (e.g. polylactic acid could be dissolved into dichloromethane), and then the solution is cast into a mold filled with porogen particles. Such porogen can be an inorganic salt like sodium chloride, crystals of saccharose, gelatin spheres or paraffin spheres. The size of the porogen particles will affect the size of the scaffold pores, while the polymer to porogen ratio is directly correlated to the amount of porosity of the final structure. After the polymer solution has been cast the solvent is allowed to fully evaporate, then the composite structure in the mold is immersed in a bath of a liquid suitable for dissolving the porogen: water in case of sodium chloride, saccharose and gelatin or an aliphatic solvent like hexane for paraffin. Once the porogen has been fully dissolved, a porous structure is obtained. Other than the small thickness range that can be obtained, another drawback of SCPL lies in its use of organic solvents which must be fully removed to avoid any possible damage to the cells seeded on the scaffold.

- *Gas foaming*: To overcome the necessity to use organic solvents and solid porogens a technique using gas as a porogen has been developed. First disk shaped structures made of the desired polymer are prepared by means of compression molding using a heated mold. The disks are then placed in a chamber where are exposed to high pressure $CO_2$ for several days. The pressure inside the chamber is gradually restored to atmospheric levels.

During this procedure the pores are formed by the carbon dioxide molecules that abandon the polymer, resulting in a sponge like structure. The main problems related to such a technique are caused by the excessive heat used during compression molding (which prohibits the incorporation of any temperature labile material into the polymer matrix) and by the fact that the pores do not form an interconnected structure.

- *Emulsification/Freeze-drying*: This technique does not require the use of a solid porogen like SCPL. First a synthetic polymer is dissolved into a suitable solvent (e.g. polylactic acid in dichloromethane) then water is added to the polymeric solution and the two liquids are mixed in order to obtain an emulsion. Before the two phases can separate, the emulsion is cast into a mold and quickly frozen by means of immersion into liquid nitrogen. The frozen emulsion is subsequently freeze-dried to remove the dispersed water and the solvent, thus leaving a solidified, porous polymeric structure. While emulsification and freeze-drying allows a faster preparation if compared to SCPL, since it does not require a time consuming leaching step, it still requires the use of solvents, moreover pore size is relatively small and porosity is often irregular. Freeze-drying by itself is also a commonly employed technique for the fabrication of scaffolds. In particular it is used to prepare collagen sponges: collagen is dissolved into acidic solutions of acetic acid or hydrochloric acid that are cast into a mold, frozen with liquid nitrogen then liophylized.

- *Liquid-liquid phase separation*: Similar to the previous technique, this procedure requires the use of a solvent with a low melting point that is easy to sublime. For example, dioxane could be used to dissolve polylactic acid, then phase separation is induced through the addition of a small quantity of water: a polymer-rich and a polymer-poor phase are formed. Following cooling below the solvent melting point and some days of vacuum-drying to sublime the solvent a porous scaffold is obtained. Liquid-liquid phase separation presents the same drawbacks of emulsification/freeze-drying.

- *CAD/CAM technologies*: Since most of the above described approaches are limited when it comes to the control of porosity and pore size, computer assisted design and manufacturing techniques have been introduced to tissue engineering. First a three-dimensional structure is designed using CAD software, and then the scaffold is realized by using ink-jet printing of polymer powders or through Fused Deposition Modeling of a polymer melt **(Fig. 6.7)**.

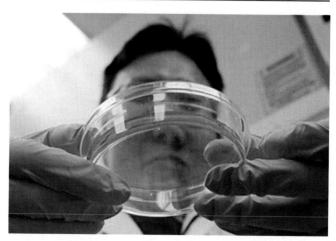

Fig. 6.7: Stem cells placed in a culture dish

## ASSEMBLY METHODS

One of the continuing, persistent problems with tissue engineering is mass transport limitations. Engineered tissues generally lack an initial blood supply, thus making it difficult for any implanted cells to obtain sufficient oxygen and nutrients to survive, and/or function properly.

Self-assembly may play an important role here, both from the perspective of encapsulating cells and proteins, as well as creating scaffolds on the right physical scale for engineered tissue constructs and cellular in growth.

It might be possible to print organs, or possibly entire organisms. A recent innovative method of construction uses an ink-jet mechanism to print precise layers of cells in a matrix of thermoreversible gel. Endothelial cells, the cells that line blood vessels, have been printed in a set of stacked rings. When incubated, these fused into a tube **(Fig. 6.8)**.

## BIOMATERIAL SUBSTRATES FOR CLONAL EXPANSION OF GENETICALLY ENGINEERED STEM CELLS

An important potential clinical application of stem cells is their use in cell replacement therapy for inherited genetic disorders. Using viral vector transduction, stem cells can be manipulated *in vitro* to correct genetic aberrations or deficiencies. When transplanted into patients, such cells might restore normal tissue function. As the sites of viral vector insertion are largely random in distribution, there is a risk of neoplastic transformation of individual transduced clones. This risk may, however, be managed by the safe design of viral vectors. Alternatively, a preselection step for clones that do not harbor deleterious insertions, followed by a thorough preclinical evaluation of these clones in

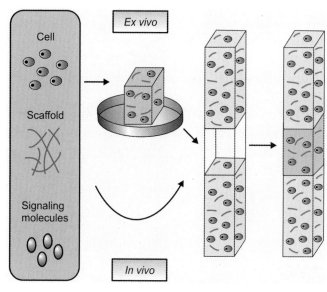

**Fig. 6.8:** Tissue engineering

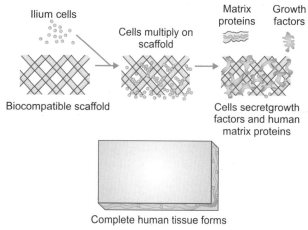

**Fig. 6.9:** Tissue engineering using stem cells

animals, may minimize the risk. *Ex vivo* expansion of preselected clones can be achieved in a bioreactor fabricated from a suitable biomaterial to produce sufficient cells to engraft a patient.

## BIOMATERIALS FOR DIFFERENTIATION OF STEM CELLS

The plasticity of ESCs represents a proverbial double-edged sword for its use in clinical application. Although clearly a desirable property owing to the tremendous differentiation repertoire that it accords, it also poses a risk of tumorigenicity. Undifferentiated cells that retain pluripotency give rise to tumors known as teratomas. Hence, it is critical for any therapeutic strategy employing a stem cell-based approach to ensure complete and irreversible differentiation of stem cells into the desired progenitors or terminal target cell type. This may be accomplished by supplementing the appropriate trophic factors in the culture medium, or delivering them from a scaffold in a controlled manner **(Fig. 6.9)**.

Different technologies have been developed to incorporate drug delivery function into a scaffold. Proteins, peptides, or plasmid DNA can be loaded into microspheres and uniformly dispersed in a macroporous polymeric scaffold, or they can be encapsulated in a fiber before forming a fibrous scaffold. This biomaterials-based approach to provide a local and sustained delivery of growth factors would be particularly valuable for the tissue development of ES-seeded scaffolds *in vivo*. The mechanical properties of a scaffold or culture surface can also exert significant influence on the differentiation of the seeded stem cell. By exerting traction

forces on a substrate, many mature cell types such as epithelial cells, fibroblasts, muscle cells, and neurons sense the stiffness of the substrate and show dissimilar morphology and adhesive characteristics. This mechanosensitivity has recently been extended to the differentiation of MSCs. When cultured on agarose gels with increasing cross-linking densities, human MSCs differentiated into neuronal, muscle, or bone lineages according to the stiffness of the matrix which approximated that of brain, muscle, and bone tissue, respectively. Highlighting the importance of matrix elasticity in dictating stem cell fate, this study also suggests an interesting biomaterial approach to influence the differentiation of stem cells **(Figs 6.10A and B)**.

## BIOMATERIALS AS CELL CARRIERS FOR *IN VIVO* STEM CELL DELIVERY

The loss of implanted cells can arise due to cytotoxicity or failure of the cells to integrate into host tissue, which presents a significant challenge to current approaches to tissue regeneration. Sites of injury or diseased organs often present hostile environments for healthy cells to establish and repopulate owing to the heightened immunological surveillance and the high concentration of inflammatory cytokines at these sites. Therefore, an additional role for TE scaffolds is to insulate their cellular cargos from the host immune system, obviating the need for a harsh immunosuppressive regime to promote the survival of grafts. Alginate-based biomaterials have been found to immunoprotect encapsulated cells and preliminary studies have demonstrated their feasible use as a vehicle for stem cell delivery. The incorporation of immunomodulatory molecules into biomaterial designs may represent another strategy to tackle the issue of immunorejection.

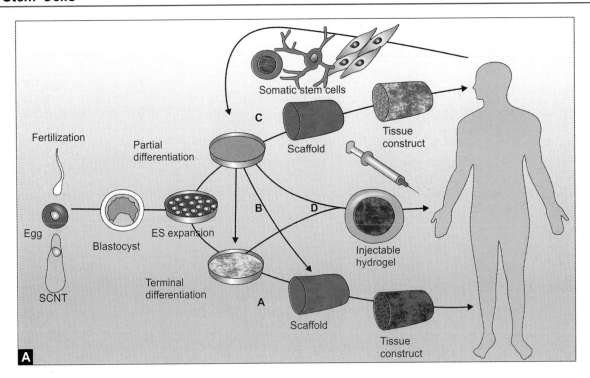

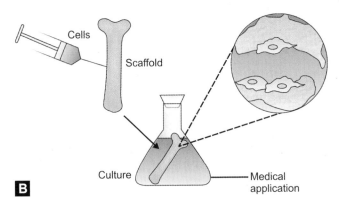

**Figs 6.10A and B:** Multiple roles for biomaterials in stem cell tissue engineering

## EMERGING TRENDS IN STEM CELL TISSUE ENGINEERING

### Micro/nanopatterned Biomaterials to Direct Stem Cell Differentiation

The influence of surface features or topography on cellular growth, movement, and orientation has long been recognized. Basement membranes, which serve as the basic substrata for cellular structures throughout the vertebrate body, are not smooth structures but, rather, are covered with grooves, ridges, pits, pores, and the fibrillar meshwork of the ECM, composed predominantly of intertwined collagen and elastin fibers with diameters ranging from 10 to 300 nm. Besides providing tensile strength and mechanical rigidity to the basement membrane, the fibrillar meshwork of protein fibers along with glycosaminoglycans also furnish binding sites for the less abundant cell-adhesion molecules. Natural stem cell niches, such as the bone marrow compartment, are replete with instructive ECM molecules secreted by stromal cells. The ECM is, however, not a completely amorphous entity but one that possesses a certain degree of quaternary organization. ECM fibers are arranged in semialigned arrays with which cells interact. At the tissue level, ordered topographical organization is more evident. For example, parallel-aligned fibrils are found in tendon, ligaments and muscles. Concentric whorls are observed in bone, and mesh-like and orthogonal lattices are present in the skin and cornea, respectively. Therefore, it is not unexpected that cells respond to topographical cues **(Fig. 6.11)**.

Studies revealed that not only are the dimensions of the topographical features important, but also their conformation—whether they are ridges, grooves, whorls, pits, pores, or steps and, more intriguingly, even their symmetry. The advent of micro- and nanofabrication technologies has made it possible to take apart and study independently the topographical and biochemical contribution to the cellular microenvironmental niche. Using technologies borrowed directly from the semiconductor and microelectronics industries, a plethora of techniques has been developed for creating patterned surfaces to investigate cellular behavior as diverse as cell–matrix and cell–cell interactions, polarized cell adhesion, cell differentiation in response to surface texture, cell migration, mechanotransduction, and cell response to gradient effects of surface-bound ligands.

Patterning techniques, such as chemical vapor deposition, physical vapor deposition, electrochemical deposition, soft lithography, photolithography, electron-beam lithography, electrospinning, layer-by-layer microfluidic patterning, three-dimensional (3D) printing, ion milling, and reactive ion etching, have been reviewed in detail by several authors. These techniques, coupled with computer aided design tools and rapid prototyping technologies, have opened up the possibility to tailor TE scaffolds with precisely controlled geometry, texture, porosity, and rigidity.

Micro- and nanoscale patterning techniques are particularly suitable for probing stem cell interaction with their microenvironment because they allow for levels of precision compatible with the delicate regulatory control of stem cell fates. Osteoblasts have proved to be a convenient model for studying cell–topography interaction as they are overtly responsive to gross topography of biomaterials.

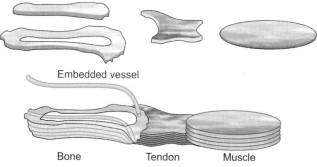

Embedded vessel

Bone          Tendon          Muscle

**Fig. 6.11:** Biomaterials in stem cell engineering

Osteoblasts displayed anisotropic behavior when cultured on nanopatterned grooves fabricated on a polystyrene surface, using a combination of Langmuir–Blodgett lithography and nanoimprinting, or on micropatterned grooves using hot embossing imprint lithography. Cells were observed to align, elongate, and migrate parallel to the grooves. The depth of the grooves was found to influence the alignment of the cells, with 150 nm grooves inducing a statistically higher degree of alignment compared to 50 nm grooves. Expression of an osteoblastic phenotype was most prominent on patterned surfaces deposited with calcium phosphate, highlighting the synergy between topography and surface chemistry. Fibrinogen coating on microgrooved surfaces fabricated from a biodegradable blend of poly (3-hydroxybutyrate-co-3-hydroxyvalerate) and poly (L/D, L-lactic acid)-enhanced osteoblast alignment along the grooves. Micropatterning of the ubiquitous.

RGDS adhesive peptide, as well as the osteoblast-specific KRSR peptide, produced ordered arrays of adhered osteoblasts. Given the responsiveness of osteoblasts to topography, it is not surprising that the success of integration of endosseous implants is dependent on their surface topography.

Substrate patterning holds particular utility in neural TE because repair of neurological injuries often requires directional guidance in terms of neuronal growth, migration, neurite projection, or synapse formation. Adult hippocampal progenitor cells (HPCs), cocultured with postnatal rat type-1 astrocytes, and extended axially along the grooves of micro patterned polystyrene substrates chemically modified with laminin. Directionally aligned poly (L-lactide) (PLLA) nanofibrous scaffolds fabricated by electrospinning induced neural stem cells (NSCs) to align themselves parallel to the fibers. Microcontact printing of neuron-adhesive peptides using poly (dimethylsiloxane) soft-lithography provides a valuable tool for studying axonal guidance and neurite formation in developmental neurobiology. TE of skeletal muscle could also potentially benefit from micro- and nanopatterning technologies. Skeletal muscle is a highly organized structure consisting of long parallel bundles of multinucleated myotubes that are formed by differentiation and fusion of myoblast satellite cells. Under normal culture conditions, on conventional tissue culture polystyrene, myoblasts grow in monolayers with fibroblastic morphology. However, in the presence of organized topographical cues, such as aligned nanofibers or micropatterned substrates, myoblasts fuse and assemble into elongated myotubes.

## SCAFFOLD-BASED NANOPARTICLE DELIVERY SYSTEM

Nanotechnology has provided new ways for functionalizing TE scaffolds with bioactive factors (drugs, proteins, or nucleic acids). Rather than doping the factors directly into the bulk material during scaffold fabrication, these factors can first be encapsulated in nanoparticles that are then dispersed into the bulk material. The factors are delivered to cells when the nanoparticles are released during scaffold degradation.

Such a delivery system offers several advantages:

- By prudent selection of nanoparticle shell material, the rate of factor release can be more tightly regulated because encapsulation in nanoparticles can limit diffusion. The rate of factor release would depend on the degradation rate of the scaffold, the size and density of the nanoparticles, as well as the nature of the nanoparticles;
- The factors can be protected from external degradation before delivery to cells, which is important for labile agents such as growth factors, plasmid DNA, and siRNA.
- Encapsulation in nanoparticles can resolve solvent incompatibility issues between the cargo and the scaffold bulk material.

## THE DEVELOPMENT OF BIOMATERIALS FOR STEM CELL EXPANSION AND DIFFERENTIATION

### ESCs

#### Expansion of ESCs

Until recently, the expansion of human ESCs was performed exclusively on feeder cell layers. However, recent reports of defined, feeder-free formulations for the derivation and maintenance of human ESCs promise to change this scenario. Biomaterials-based expansion of human ESCs has now become a distinct possibility, as has large-scale culture of human ESCs in bioreactors. This will hopefully lead to the alleviation, if not elimination, of the two major obstacles to the widespread implementation of ES technologies in the clinic, which are concerns about exposure to animal components as well as consistency in both the quality and quantity of cell supply.

Biomaterials-based expansion has been achieved with murine ESCs. A number of studies described the use of hydrogel polymers as a support substrate for the maintenance of murine ESCs and embryoid body (EB) formation.

Harrison et al evaluated the effects of modified aliphatic poly ($\alpha$-hydroxyesters) such as poly (D, L-lactide), PLLA, poly (glycolide), and PLGA on murine ESC propagation in leukemia-inhibitory factor-conditioned media. Alkali treatment of the substrate surface, which cleaves the polyester backbone to present carboxyl and hydroxyl groups, increases hydrophilicity and significantly increases the proliferation of mature ESCs.

Murine ESCs cultured on electrospun nanofibrillar polyamide matrix (Ultra-Web) showed greatly enhanced proliferation and self-renewal compared to culture on two-dimensional tissue culture surfaces, highlighting the effects of 3D topography. Molecular analysis of the cultured cells revealed the activation of the small GTPase Rac, and the phosphoinositide 3-kinase pathway, which are both associated with stem cell self-renewal and upregulation of Nanog, a homeoprotein required for maintenance of pluripotency. It was postulated that the 3D microarchitecture of Ultraweb mimicked the ECM/basement membrane so as to activate stem cell proliferation and self-renewal.

Human ESCs have been expanded *in vitro* as cell aggregates known as EBs. Culture of human ESCs in a slow-turning lateral vessel bioreactor yielded up to a threefold increase in EB formation compared to static dish cultures. Subsequently, the formation of human EBs within a 3D porous alginate scaffolds was reported. There is, however, a tendency for cultured human EBs to undergo spontaneous differentiation, particularly vasculogenesis. A good understanding of the factors affecting ESC self-renewal and maintenance and the underlying gene regulatory and signal transduction mechanisms will be instrumental in directing future designs of biomaterials for ES expansion.

#### Differentiation of Embryonic Stem Cells (ESCs)

Achieving production of specific tissues from ESCs will require precise control of their differentiation. This would involve both physical and biochemical cues acting in concert. The versatility of such a concept was demonstrated by the induction of human with ESC differentiation into distinct embryonic tissue types within a biodegradable 3D polymer scaffold made from a 50:50 blend of PLGA and PLLA. The type of tissue produced depended on the differentiation growth factor that was supplemented. Retinoic acid and transforming growth factor $\alpha$ induced ESC differentiation into 3D structures with characteristics of developing neural tissues and cartilage, respectively, whereas activin-A or insulin-like growth factor induced liver-like tissues.

Although cell seeding was carried out in the presence of Matrigel or onto scaffolds precoated with fibronectin, it was shown that neither Matrigel nor fibronectin alone could potentiate the effects observed with the PLGA/PLLA scaffolds. It was therefore hypothesized that the mechanical stiffness conferred by the scaffold acted synergistically with the Matrigel or fibronectin to enhance human ESC differentiation and 3D organization. Furthermore, it was shown that tissue constructs made with the scaffolds integrated well into host tissues when transplanted into severe combined immunodeficiency (SCID) mice. Supplementation of retinoic acid, nerve growth factor, or neurotropin 3 induced neural rosette-like structures throughout the scaffolds. Nerve growth factor and neurotropin 3 induced the expression of nestin, a marker of neural precursor cells, as well as the formation of vascular structures. Pure PLLA scaffold was a suitable carrier for *in vivo* mineralization of human ESCs in SCID mice.

## Hematopoietic Stem Cells (HSCs)

Despite almost three decades of extensive research into HSC expansion and self-renewal, a stable and reliable expansion system for human HSCs has yet to be achieved. This is probably due to the extreme sensitivity of true HSCs to their immediate micromilieu. Minute fluctuations in cytokine concentrations, oxygen tension, temperature, and cell–ECM interactions are sufficient to set in motion irreversible differentiation cascades that lead to depletion of HSCs in culture. Stroma- and cytokine-free expansion of HSCs/hematopoietic progenitor cells (HPCs) using a porous biocompatible 3D scaffold was first described by Bagley et al

Scaffolds fabricated from tantalum-coated porous biomaterials (TCPB matrix or Cellfoam) presented a microarchitecture reminiscent of bone marrow trabeculae. Culture of bone marrow HPC on TCPB in the absence of cytokine augmentation maintained progenitor phenotype and multipotency up to 6 weeks; a considerably longer period compared them with cultures grown on fibronectin-coated plastic dishes, bone marrow stroma cocultures, and other 3D devices. In particular, culture on TCPB matrix led to a 1.5-fold expansion of HPC numbers following 1 week in culture and a 6.7-fold increases in colony-forming ability following 6 weeks in culture.

Supplementation with low concentration (ng/ml) of stem cell factor and Flt3-ligand, but not interleukin 3, markedly enhanced the effects of TCPB matrix in maintaining the multipotency of HPCs. The use of low concentrations of cytokines in *ex vivo* expansion of HSCs/HPCs has clinical relevance as it has been shown that exposure of these cells to high, nonphysiological levels of cytokines before transplantation diminishes their ability to engraft into bone marrow. Improved expansion outcome was also observed for cord blood-derived CD34+ cells cultured on TCPB scaffolds. Culture on TCPB scaffold for 2 weeks yielded a threefold increase in the number of nucleated cells and a 2.6-fold increased in colony-forming units. Both CD45+ and CD34+ cells increased threefold in number. Additionally, expanded cells were capable of engrafting sublethally irradiated, nonobese diabetic/SCID mice.

More recently, the effects of surface-immobilized cell adhesive peptides and polypeptides on the proliferation and differentiation of purified cord blood CD34+ cells were investigated. Fibronectin covalently grafted onto 3D poly (ethylene terephthalate) (PET) nonwoven scaffolds markedly improved the maintenance of the CD34+ phenotype, multipotency, and nonobese diabetic/SCID engraftment efficiency of cultured cord blood CD34+ progenitor cells compared to fibronectin-grafted two-dimensional scaffolds or tissue culture plastic controls. It was hypothesized that immobilized fibronectin synergized with the 3D topography of the modified scaffolds to create a biomimetic microenvironment for CD34+ proliferation and maintenance. Purified cord blood CD34+ HSCs cultured in reconstituted collagen I fibrils in the presence of Flt3-ligand, stem cell factor, and interleukin 3 for 7 days of culture showed increased number of colony-forming units, although the total expansion factor of CD34+ cells was slightly lower compared to control suspension cultures, suggesting that collagen I scaffold performed better at preserving the multipotency of the CD34+ cells. Gene-expression profiling of the cultured cells revealed the upregulation of more than 50 genes in the presence of collagen I. Among these, genes for several growth factors, cytokines, and chemokines (*e.g.* interleukin 8 and macrophage inhibitory protein 1α) were confirmed using quantitative polymerase chain reaction. In addition, higher expression of the negative cell-cycle regulator BTG2/TIS21 and an inhibitor of the mitogen-activated protein kinase pathway, DUSP2, underline the regulatory role of the ECM. Together, these data show that the expansion of CD34+ cord blood cells in a culture system containing a 3D collagen I matrix induces a qualitative change in the gene expression profile of cultivated HSCs.

## Mesenchymal Stem Cells (MSCs)

### Mesenchymal Stem Cells Expansion

Mesenchymal stem cells have been extensively studied for TE owing to their potential to differentiate into osteogenic, chondrogenic, and adipogenic tissues, which are major targets for reparative medicine. In addition, recent evidence demonstrated their potential for neural transdifferentiation both *in vitro* and *in vivo*, and for differentiation into smooth muscle cells. Adherence to tissue culture plastic has been used as a criterion for selection of MSCs from other cell types during their purification from bone marrow and umbilical cord blood. Although tissue culture plastic could support extensive proliferation of MSCs, continuing efforts are being made to develop an optimal substrate for MSC expansion. Clinical scale expansion of MSCs is achievable using bioreactor culture.

### MSC Differentiation

Although much has been learned about the roles of biological factors in inducing MSCs differentiation, the roles played by the physical environment in this process are only emerging. Surface chemistries of substrates alone appear sufficient to alter the differentiation of MSCs. Although unmodified and modified silane surfaces supported MSC maintenance, –NH2- and –SH-modified surfaces promoted osteogenic differentiation, and –COOH- and –OH-modified surfaces promoted chondrogenic differentiation. Mechanical signals such as local stresses (tensile, compressive, shear), geometry, topography, and cell–cell contact have a direct influence on the differentiation of MSCs. McBeath et al. demonstrated that the fate of MSCs differentiation can be altered by manipulating cell shape using a micropatterned adhesive substrate. Enforced spherical cell morphology led to preferential adipogenic commitment, whereas a flattened morphology induced osteoblastic commitment. Cell shape was further shown to influence the differentiation fate via cytoskeletal mechanics, most probably transduced by RhoA signaling.

### Biomaterials for Osteogenic Differentiation of MSCs

A wide range of biomaterials has been tested to harness the osteogenic potential of MSCs for bone TE. Constituents mimicking natural bone have often been incorporated into biomaterial design to stimulate ossification. Calcium and phosphate ions are important components during the mineralization phase of the ossification process. Materials composed of calcium phosphate such as hydroxyapatite [HA; $Ca_{10}(PO_4)_6(OH)_2$] and tricalcium phosphate [TCP; $Ca_3(PO_4)_2$] are attractive candidates for bone substitutes. HA is a natural component of bone and has been clinically tested for orthopedic and periodontal applications. HA coating has been shown to improve the outcome of prosthetic implants. Porous HA ceramics supported bone formation by marrow MSCs *in vitro* and *in vivo*.

A number of unique characteristics of HA contribute to its osteoconductive property. HA is known to strongly adsorb fibronectin and vitronectin, ligands for the integrin family of cell adhesion receptors that play key roles in mediating adhesion of MSCs and osteoblast precursors. In addition, when used in blends with other polymers, HA particles exposed on the surface of scaffolds favor focal contact formation of osteoblasts. A bone-like mineral film consisting mainly of calcium apatite, when introduced onto the surface of poly (lactide-co-glycolide) substrate, could achieve the same effect as when HA was incorporated into the bulk material. It is also believed that HA degradation products create an alkaline microenvironment and provide electrolytes necessary for mineralization of ECM by osteoblasts during bone formation. This microenvironment then recruits surrounding cells to acquire an osteoblastic phenotype and to participate in the ossification process.

Composites of HA with other polymers have been evaluated as osteoconductive substrates. Scaffolds fabricated from a composite consisting of HA/chitosan gelatin promoted initial cell adhesion, supported 3.3-fold higher cellularity and could maintain higher progenicity of MSCs compared with chitosan gelatin alone. Biphasic calcium phosphate ceramics, composed of a mixture of HA and $\alpha$-tricalcium phosphate are considered to be more bioactive and more efficient than HA alone for the repair of periodontal defects and certain orthopedic applications. A macroporous form of biphasic calcium phosphate can promote bone formation and has a degradation rate compatible with bone in growth kinetics. Mineralized collagen sponges constructed of cross-linked collagen-1 fibers coated with noncrystal HA improved cell seeding and induced osteogenic differentiation of human MSCs. When seeded with fibrinogen hydrogel into a polycaprolactone-HA composite scaffold, human MSCs differentiated efficiently into osteoblasts under osteogenic medium conditions.

Other forms of calcium phosphate-containing material that have been assessed for osteoconductivity are octacalcium phosphate and $\alpha$-tricalcium phosphate. Tissue constructs of various conformations including two-dimensional cell sheets and 3D blocks were achieved with rat MSCs seeded on octacalcium phosphate crystal micro-scaffolds. Macroporous $\alpha$-TCP was demonstrated to support osteogenesis from human MSCs. Bioactive glass fibers possess several characteristics attractive for bone TE. Firstly, they spontaneously initiate precipitation of HA on their surface, which renders them osteoconductive. Secondly, their fibrillar nature mimics the porosity of bone material and also the fibrillar organization of collagen fibrils that are orthogonally distributed within natural bone. Bioactive glass integrated well with surrounding bone tissue when used as defect fillers.

Composites of bioactive glass with other biodegradable polymers, such as phospholipase, facilitated the formation of crystalline HA on the surface, which was conducive for MSC proliferation and differentiation into osteoblasts. Bone ECM components profoundly influence the activity of MSCs. Bone matrix consists primarily of fibronectin, collagen types I and IV, laminin, and the glycosaminoglycans heparin sulfate, chondroitin sulfate, and hyaluronan. Recent evidence suggests that the different response of MSCs to different 3D polymeric scaffolds may be determined by the adsorptivity of the polymer for various ECM components present in the culture medium. For example, polycapro-lactone mediates MSC attachment primarily via adsorbed vitronectin, whereas PLGA does so via adsorbed type-I collagen. Incorporation of these components into bone TE scaffolds provides a way to control the behavior of MSCs more precisely. Scaffolds composed of hyaluronan, a major glycosaminoglycan found in bone ECM, have been demons-trated to modulate the expression of molecules associated with the inflammatory response as well as that of bone remodeling metalloproteinases and their inhibitors by human MSCs. This finding has a significant impact on the construction of bone grafts for clinical use. Human MSCs cultured on a poly (3-hydroxybutyrate) fabric scaffold, immobilized with chondroitin sulfate, displayed phenotype and gene expression consistent with extensive osteogenesis. Honeycomb collagen scaffolds fabricated from bovine dermal atelocollagen provided a superior surface for MSC proliferation and osteoblastic differentiation compared to a tissue culture plastic control.

## Biomaterials for Chondrogenic Differentiation of MSCs

Conventional TE of cartilage suffers from an inadequate supply of autologous chondrocytes. Deriving chondrocytes from MSCs has become an attractive alternative. A wide spectrum of natural and synthetic biomaterials has been investigated for chondrogenic differentiation of MSCs. Several studies have described the use of natural polymers such as silk, cellulose, hyaluronan, hyaluronic acid, agarose, and marine sponge fiber skeleton. In addition, hybrid polymers, composed of synthetic and natural polymer blends, or of different natural polymers and their derivatives, have been tested. For example, (PLGA)-gelatin/chondroitin/hyaluronate scaffolds proved to be superior as a carrier of autologous MSCs in repairing full-thickness cartilage defects in rabbits compared with PLGA scaffolds. Cho et al developed an injectable thermosensitive hydrogel from a copolymer of water-soluble chitosan and Poly (*N*-isopropylacrylamide) (WSC-*g*-PNIPAAm) for chondrogenic differentiation of human MSCs. When injected into the submucosal layer of the bladder of rabbits, cells entrapped in the copolymer underwent further chondrogenesis and formed tissue resembling articular cartilage composed of a mixture of hyaline and fibrous cartilage and other tissue components.

Electrospun polycaprolactone nanofibrous scaffold has proven to be an interesting substrate for chondrogenic differentiation of MSCs. Richardson et al demonstrated the potential of a biodegradable PLLA scaffold as a chondroactive substrate for MSCs-based TE of intervertebral disks. They had shown earlier that contact coculture of chondrocyte-like cells from the nucleus pulposus of the human intervertebral disk with MSCs could recruit MSCs to differentiate into nucleus pulposus cells. Guo et al. reported repair of large articular cartilage defects with implants of autologous MSCs seeded onto $\alpha$-TCP scaffolds in an ovine model.

## Neural Stem Cells (NSCs)

In mammals, adult neurons lose their proliferative potential. The central nervous system, therefore, has limited regenerative capacity when inflicted with lesions resulting from trauma, stroke, or neuropathological conditions. Clinical trials using transplantation of fetal brain cells to treat neurodegenerative diseases such as Parkinson's disease has raised questions regarding the effectiveness of this strategy. Repair of neurological injuries in the central nervous system is complicated by the presence of natural inhibitors of nerve regeneration, notably neurite outgrowth inhibitor and myelin-associated glycoprotein. Thus, a subset of therapeutic strategies for spinal cord injury is focused primarily on creating a permissive environment for regeneration by targeting these inhibitory proteins.

The peripheral nervous system retains limited capacity for self-repair if the injuries are small. Larger injuries, however, require nerve grafts usually harvested from other parts of the body. TE using NSCs provides a viable and practical alternative for cell therapy of the central nervous system and peripheral nervous system. However, there is a critical need for technologies to expand NSCs on a large scale before their use in the clinic can become commonplace. In the mammalian brain, NSCs originate from two specific regions, the subventricular zone and the dentate gyrus area of the hippocampus. Evidence suggests that NSCs are widely distributed in the adult brain **(Fig. 6.12)**. In addition, reprogramming of oligodendrocyte precursors and astrocytes could also give rise to multipotent NSCs. Recently; directed differentiation of human ESCs and MSCs into neuronal lineages has emerged as an alternative source of cells for neural TE and neuroscience research.

Pioneering work on large-scale culture of human NSCs was performed in suspension bioreactors. However, nutrient and oxygen transfer constraints limit the size of NSC aggregates, known as neurospheres, which form in suspension cultures. Propagation of NSCs in static cultures was achieved in the presence of basic fibroblast growth factor and/or epidermal growth factor, but passaging of the cells necessitated continuous mechanical dissociation of neurospheres. Many surgical procedures for treating brain lesions such as tumor and blood clot removal result in volume loss, creating cavities that should ideally are filled if recovery of neuronal integrity is desired. In addition, neurodegenerative diseases and hypoxic–ischemic injuries lead to necrotic and/or scar tissue formation that occludes normal cognitive and motor functions. Restoration of these functions would necessitate replacing the necrotic or scar tissue with healthy cells, a futuristic concept known as reconstructive brain surgery.

Successful delivery and incorporation of NSCs for cell replacement therapy of the brain hinges upon the use of a suitable carrier material. Similarly, the repair of transected spinal cord or peripheral nerve injuries with engineered grafts would depend upon proper selection of an ideal nerve conduit to bridge the injury site. Of the different types of biomaterials, resorbable polymers appear to be the most suitable candidates to fulfill these roles. Encouraging results from several studies raised optimism about the potential of neural TE in clinical applications. Using a biodegradable blend of 50:50 PLGA and a block copolymer of PLGA-polylysine, Teng et al fabricated a bilayered scaffold with outer and inner microarchitectures to mimic the white and gray matter of the spinal cord, respectively. The inner layer was seeded with NSCs and the construct was inserted into a laterally hemisected lesion of the rat spinal cord.

Animals implanted with the scaffold-NSC constructs displayed improved recovery of hindlimb locomotor functions compared with empty scaffold and cells only controls. The recovery was attributed to a reduction in tissue loss from secondary injury processes, diminished glial scarring and, to a certain extent, re-establishment of axonal connectivity across the lesion supported by the scaffold-NSC construct. An interesting finding was that an implanted poly (glycolide)-based scaffold-NSC construct could establish bidirectional feedback interactions with the brain in a reciprocal manner to mediate repair of an ischemia-induced lesion. It is worth mentioning that a novel self-assembling peptide nanofiber scaffold implanted alone without cell cargo could support axonal regeneration through the site of an acute brain injury and could restore functional neuronal connectivity in the severed optic tract in animal models. A self-assembling peptide nanofibrous scaffold, functionalized with a high density of the neurite-promoting laminin epitope, IKVAV, could rapidly induce differentiation of seeded neural progenitor cells into neurons, but at the same time suppressed the development of astrocytes. In another study, rat neural progenitor cells entrapped in a 3D collagen matrix rapidly expanded and spontaneously differentiated into excitable neurons and formed synapses. Porous foam

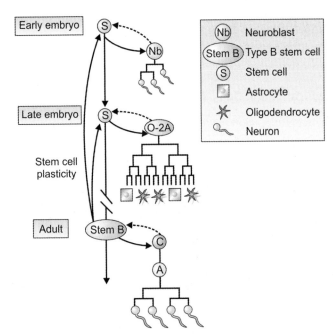

**Fig. 6.12:** Neural stem cell progeny can reacquire stem cell properties

matrices prepared from poly (styrene/divinylbenzene), using a high internal phase emulsion templating and coated with poly (D-lysine) or laminin, promoted neurite outgrowth from human embryonal carcinoma stem cell-derived neurons.

## Endothelial Progenitor Cells

Neovasculogenesis or the formation of blood vessels post-natally, is now thought to be attributed mainly to the activity of endothelial progenitor cells (EPCs). Ever since their isolation from peripheral blood mononuclear cells was first reported, EPCs have been identified from various sources including bone marrow, umbilical cord blood, vessel walls, and fetal liver. Resident EPC populations in bone marrow constitute a natural reservoir of cells that can be rapidly mobilized upon acute demand following major vascular insult. The potential application of EPCs for therapeutic vasculogenesis is widely recognized. Direct infusion of endothelial stem/progenitor cells from various sources for neovascularization has been evaluated extensively in preclinical and clinical studies. Early strategies for developing vascular prostheses focused on the delivery of angiogenic growth factors such as vascular endothelial growth factor, fibroblast growth factor-2, and DNA encoding these factors to induce in growth of microvessels from the host vascu-lature *in situ. In vitro* pre-endothelialization was hypothesized to create an antithrombogenic barrier for the devices, thereby preventing thrombus occlusion. Artificial grafts were seeded with differentiated endothelial cells (ECs) or ECs in combination with other cell types such as smooth muscle cells.

Owing to their undifferentiated state, EPCs retain the potential to remodel and integrate into the site at which they are transplanted. Kaushal et al implanted grafts constructed from decellularized iliac vessels preseeded with EPCs in a sheep model. EPC-seeded grafts remained patent for 130 days, whereas nonseeded grafts occluded within 15 days. Furthermore, explanted EPC grafts exhibited contractile activity and nitric oxide-mediated vascular relaxation that were similar to native arteries. EPCs have also been employed in intraluminal endothelialization of small-diameter metallic stents. In variations of the experiment, EPCs were used for surface endothelialization of whole metallic stents coated with a photoreactive gelatin layer or endothelialization of a small-diameter compliant graft made of microporous segmented polyurethane and coated with photoreactive gelatin. The EPC layer displayed antithrombogenic properties similar to that of mature ECs. EPC-endothelialized small diameter compliant grafts, molded from type-I collagen

and strengthened with segmented polyurethane film, remained patent for up to 3 months in a canine implantation model.

Living tissue patches comprising umbilical cord myofibroblasts and EPCs seeded on poly (glycolide)/P4HB mesh scaffolds have been fabricated for potential application in pediatric cardiovascular repair. Fibrin coating of polymer scaffolds has been shown to promote the attachment of EPCs. Mature ECs derived from cord blood EPCs have also been explored for endothelialization of vascular grafts. Recent scaffold fabrication techniques, in particular aligned, coaxial electrospinning holds particular promise for the engineering of vascular grafts. In addition to providing a surface texture ideal for cell attachment and alignment, combinations of polymers can be selected to recapitulate the viscoelastic properties of natural vessels as well as to selectively promote the growth of EPCs and smooth muscles cells to generate a more biomimetic graft.

## Embryonic Germ Cell–Derived Primordial Germ Cells

Human embryonic germ (EG) cells are a potential alternative to ESCs as a source of pluripotent stem cells for cell therapy and regenerative medicine. EG cells are derived by the adaptation of primordial germ cells to survive and self-renew in culture. Despite the lower ethical acceptance of EGs owing to their controversial origin and the difficulty of maintaining well defined EG lines *in vitro*, there is evidence to suggest that they follow a different epigenetic program than ESCs, and this may accentuate their importance as an alternative stem cell source in the future. Thus far, only a limited number of studies have investigated the potential use of EGs for TE. Yim and Leong reported evidence of neuronal differentiation of EG-derived EBs cultured on a cellulose acetate nanofibrous scaffold surface-decorated with nerve growth factor.

Culture on a biodegradable scaffold, composed of poly (epsilon-caprolactone-co-ethyl ethylene phosphate) and unmodified cellulose acetate, led to enhanced proliferation of EBs. Extended culture (10 months) on the two scaffolds produced cellular outcomes, with EBs cultured on poly (epsilon-caprolactone-co-ethyl ethylene phosphate) scaffold secreting copious amounts of ECM while showing down-regulation of the expression of neural markers. This study highlighted the fact that the architecture and biodegradability of the scaffolds play an important role in determining the fate of EG cells in cell culture.

## Adipose Tissue Derived Stem Cells

Adipose tissue derived stem cells (ADSCs) display much the same surface markers as bone marrow derived MSCs with the exception of the presence of VLA-4 expression and the absence of the expression of its receptor, CD106. Consistent with this phenotypic similarity, the two cell types exhibit an almost indistinguishable differentiation repertoire. Under suitable culture conditions, ADSCs differentiate along classical mesenchymal lineages, namely adipogenesis, chondrogenesis, osteogenesis, and myogenesis. Interest in ADSCs lies primarily in their potential as an alternative to bone marrow MSCs. Although they occur at frequencies comparable to those of their bone marrow counterparts, the extraction protocol for ADSCs is deemed less invasive than that for bone marrow harvests. Additionally, these cells may prove valuable in treating conditions associated with bone marrow failure.

The capacity of ADSC to differentiate along various lineages, when seeded into polymeric scaffolds, has been evaluated both *in vitro* and *in vivo*. In an attempt to find the minimal sequence of laminin sufficient to promote ADSC attachment on TE scaffolds, Santiago et al covalently immobilized RGD, YIGSR, and IKVAV peptide sequences on a polycaprolactone surface. ADSCs were found to adhere most avidly to an IKVAV-modified surface. ADSCs cultured on scaffolds formed by agglomeration of chitosan particles, showed evidence of osteogenic and chondrogenic differentiation. Encapsulation in agarose hydrogels and gelatin scaffolds was permissive for chondrogenic differentiation of ADSCs. ADSCs seeded in HA/TCP scaffolds or in collagen/HA–TCP composite matrix showed definitive osteogenesis when implanted into SCID mice. In side-by-side comparison to bone marrow MSCs, ADSCs in atelo-collagen honeycomb-shaped or β-TCP scaffolds showed no distinguishable differences in osteogenic differentiation either *in vitro* or when implanted into nude mice.

Adipose TE using ADSCs is currently being contemplated as a viable alternative strategy in plastic, corrective, and reconstructive surgery. Trials using mature autologous adipose tissue have only met with limited success because of tissue resorption and ensuing calcification. A confounding factor is that mature adipocytes are terminally differentiated and postmitotic. ADSCs is speculated to circumvent some of these drawbacks. Animal studies have provided proof-of-concept for this approach. *In vivo* adipogenesis has been demonstrated with implanted ADSCs seeded in collagen, hyaluronic acid, phospholipase, PLGA, and phospholipase/poly (glycolide) composite scaffolds. A consensus from these studies is that a polymeric scaffold is beneficial for adipose tissue formation from implanted ADSCs. In addition to classical mesenchymal lineages, ADSCs have been shown to be capable of crossing developmental boundaries and to transdifferentiate into skeletal muscle, cardiomyocytes, neurons, and ECs. Although some of these cells have been tested in scaffold-free cell therapies, their use in biomaterials-based TE offers areas for exploration.

## Other Stem/Progenitor Cells with Potential for TE Applications

A number of more recently identified stem/progenitor cells provide interesting subjects for research and are probable candidates for organ-specific TE. The recent report of the isolation of human renal progenitor cells from adult kidney is set to launch a new branch of TE. End stage renal failure is a catastrophic disease usually leading to death. Conventional treatments such as kidney transplantation and renal dialysis have severe limitations and are often associated with considerable morbidity. Although the idea of a tissue-engineered kidney is not novel, the use of renal stem cells could allow for the construction of a new organ *de novo* as well as for prospects for creating an autologous organ.

Microporous scaffolds and the implementation of microfluidic technologies could be envisaged to take the lead in this arena. TE of a functional pancreas has been an area of intense research for several decades. Multipotent adult pancreatic progenitor cells identified recently will provide momentum to make this goal achievable in the near future. Other newly discovered stem/progenitor cells that have broadened the cellular arsenal for regenerative medicine include liver, retinal, skeletal muscle, hair follicle, and dentine pulp stem cells.

## CHALLENGES TO STEM CELL TE

In spite of justified optimism, several major challenges remain to be met.

- Foremost is the problem of mass transport during scale-up of engineered tissue constructs. Any TE modality that aspires toward clinical translation must consider vascularization. This hurdle is currently viewed as the limiting factor to the size of tissue constructs that can realistically be achieved. Supply of nutrients and oxygen to cells located deep in bulk tissue or complex organs must be resolved in order for them to be maintained in the body for any meaningful duration. Thrombogenic occlusion of microconduits or micropores introduced into biomaterial constructs is a common problem faced in tackling this limitation. The incorporation of antithrombogenic molecules into biomaterials is one of the strategies employed to overcome the problem. Alternatively, angiogenic factors can be incorporated into biomaterials to induce *de novo* vasculogenesis and/or angiogenesis from tissues surrounding the implants. Spontaneous vasculogenesis observed under certain conditions, such as in human ESC EBs growing in suspension cultures lends hope to surmounting this challenge.

- Another challenge is the requirement for innervations. In fact, this requirement has been the major obstacle in the development of an implantable hybrid liver assist device. The liver is richly innervated via both the sympathetic and parasympathetic pathways from the hypothalamus and adrenal glands, which regulate functions such as blood flow through the hepatic sinusoids, solute exchange, and parenchymal function. Innervation is also required by other organs such as muscles, the pulmonary system, the kidney, and endocrine glands. Therefore, selection of biomaterials and the design of a tissue construct for repairing these organ systems would have to take into account the provision for innervations.

- Organ systems are not composed of a homogeneous cell type, but rather an assembly of different cell types either intermingled together or partitioned into discrete sublocations. Each of these cell types may have unique substratum requirements. Engineering of complex organs would, therefore, need to cater to each component cell type. A challenge remains to find the correct balance between the biological and physical properties of the scaffold material to suit each cell type. In this respect, TE using stem cells has clear advantages, because the plasticity of the cells can allow for *de novo* formation of tissues depending on scaffold composition. *In situ* remodeling at the interface between different cell types, akin to events that occur between germ layers during embryogenesis, can give rise to new tissues. This may theoretically relax the stringency for precise substratum requirements.

The creation of relevant disease models to evaluate the efficacy of the engineered tissue constructs is as important as overcoming the engineering hurdles. Often, small rodent models with mechanically or pharmacologically induced lesions do not accurately recapitulate human disease conditions, causing disparate outcomes between preclinical and clinical trials. Nonhuman primate models may, in theory, provide the most relevant animal models, but these are not readily available for practical and ethical reasons. The creation of nonhuman primate models for various human diseases by gene targeting and nuclear transfer has been proposed. However, cloning of monkeys remains unsuccessful to date. Success in this arena may positively impact stem cell TE.

## NONHUMAN PRIMATE MODELS

The use of human embryos to derive embryonic stem cells (ES cells) is viewed by some sectors of our society as ethically problematic. In nonhuman primates, there are currently three methods for deriving pluripotent stem cells: from embryos produced by:

1. *In vitro* fertilization
2. Parthenogenesis
3. Adult tissues such as cells derived from the bone marrow.

Finally the field of TE has entered an exciting new chapter, where experimental technologies are being aggressively explored for clinical translation, signifying a veritable "coming of age" of the field. The convergence of two important disciplines, that of biomaterials engineering and stem cell research, promises to revolutionize regenerative medicine. With this merger, several concepts that would have been deemed far-fetched a few years ago are now being actively pursued. Among these concepts are brain reconstructive surgery, tailor-made autologous body replacement parts, and cybernetic prosthesis. The future of stem cell TE is undoubtedly technology driven. New applications and improvement upon current designs will depend heavily on innovations in biomaterials engineering. Concomitant with this, progress in stem cell biology will be imperative in dictating advances in stem cell TE. A better understanding of the molecular mechanisms by which substrate interactions impact stem cell self-renewal and differentiation is of paramount importance for targeted design of biomaterials. Discoveries in the fields of developmental biology and functional genomics should also be parlayed for broadening the repertoire of biological molecules that can be incorporated into biomaterials for fine-tuning stem cell activities. With the merger between the two powerful disciplines biomaterials engineering and stem cell biology—a new drawing board now lies before us to develop therapies that could hopefully help the world population age more gracefully.

## TISSUE ENGINEERING AND CHARACTERIZATION

### Cartilage Tissue Engineering

Most tissues require a fully developed vascular system to oxygen and nutrients. This makes the tissues difficult to engineer, as they can die in the patient's body before they can develop a blood supply. Articular cartilage tissue, however, does not require a blood supply, acquiring its nutrients and oxygen by diffusion from its surface. Implanted cartilage does, therefore, generally survive well in the patient **(Fig. 6.13)**.

Cartilage is also a clinically important tissue, as it does not recover well from injury, and its deterioration is associated with debilitating diseases of old age, such as arthritis, which is of growing concern in the developed world. Cartilage occurs as three types within the body:

*Elastic cartilage*, an example of which is found in the ears.

*Hypertrophic cartilage* is laid down as a template for bone growth, and this may serve as a useful precursor tissue to bone (which requires a good blood supply) in tissue engineering approaches to orthopedics. Studies are underway at Sheffield to evaluate this approach to tissue engineering bone for reconstructive surgery.

*Hyaline cartilage* is found in the ribs, nasal septum and covering the bone ends of joints, such as the knees and hips. In the joints the cartilage is known as articular and is vital for cushioning and lubricating surfaces.

Research at Sheffield has focussed on evaluating the cell biology of engineered cartilage, developed using a variety of different scaffolds and growth media, and comparing this with natural material. The primary cell type in cartilage is the chondrocyte, this is a specialized cell that can survive compression and shear forces within the collagen matrix.

Histological studies have shown that the chondrocyte is embedded in a zone of specialized matrix, forming a chondron. This structure is essential to for the survival of the cell under conditions of load and shear stress. Studies have demonstrated that diseased (arthritic) chondrocytes develop a reduced chondron, and are therefore, more susceptible to damage **(Fig. 6.14)**.

### Bone Tissue Engineering

Researchers at Sheffield are pursuing two broad strategies to tackle the challenges presented by the need to engineer a

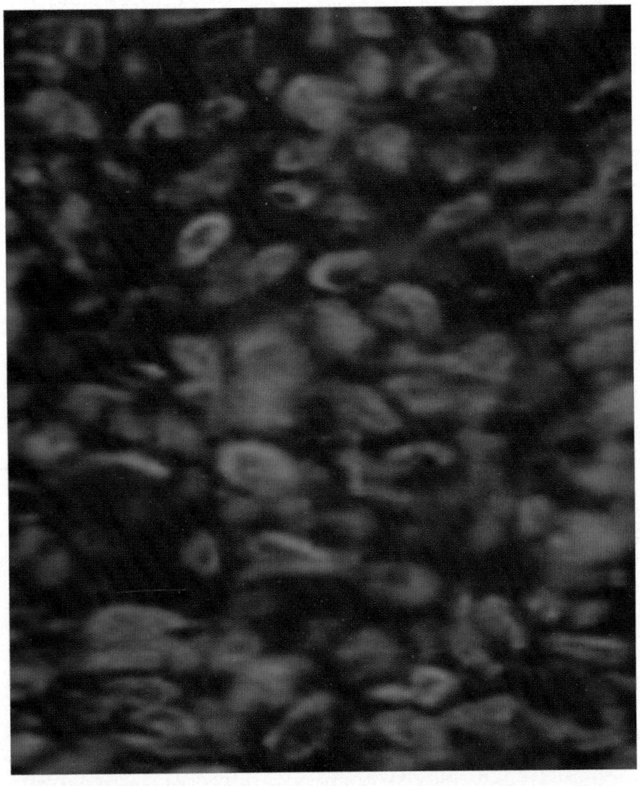

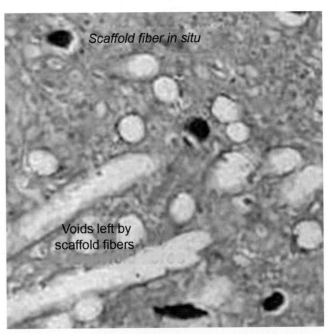

**Fig. 6.13:** Photomicrograph of engineered cartilage stained to show the specialized pericellular matrix which is important in cell signalling and protecting the chondrocyte under compressive loading

**Fig. 6.14:** Photomicrograph of engineered cartilage stained to show collagen II (orange ground). Collagen II is a vital support protein secreted by chondrocytes in natural collagen. Its appearance in this engineered tissue is indicative of a good culture regime

tissue for bone repair. Working with a local company (Ceramisys Ltd.), we are evaluating porous calcium phosphate ceramics for use as a cell support and scaffold for bone tissue engineering. Porous ceramics are seeded with mesenchymal stem cells from the bone marrow and cultured under osteogenic conditions. The resulting constructs are evaluated using a range of techniques including histology, electron microscopy, and microCT (in collaboration with Ralph Muller in Zurich as part of the EXPERTISSUES project) **(Fig. 6.15)**. Researchers are also investigating the potential of hypertrophic chondrocytes to generate a tissue engineered construct for bone repair. This approach is attractive as hypertrophic chondrocytes are able to survive with relatively little oxygen (hypoxia) such as an injury site or wound bed.

## Periodontal Tissue Engineering

The periodontal ligament forms a sheath about the root of the tooth. It acts as a shock absorber, as well as holding the tooth firmly in place. Due to the embryological development of the tooth root, however, cells in the periodontal ligament cannot regenerate **(Fig. 6.16)**.

As a consequence the ligament wears out over time in a process of chronic peridontitis, the most common cause of tooth loss, though it does not commonly manifest itself until later life. Research aims at regenerating the lost connective tissue by growing up large numbers of ligament cells and reimplanting them.

Normally cultured cells must adhere to a surface to survive and continue developing. If only presented with

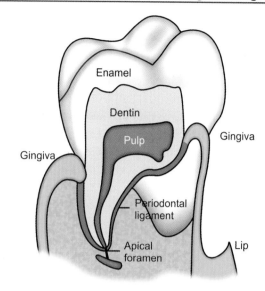

Fig. 6.16: A three-dimensional model of a human molar sectioned to show internal structure, and that of the periodontium. The periodontal ligament is depicted in pale blue

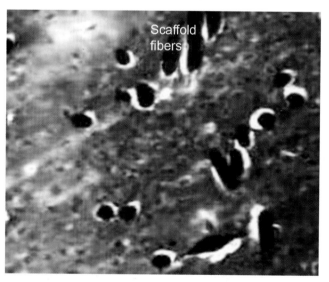

Fig. 6.17: Photomicrograph of engineered cartilage stained to show proteoglycan (purple). Proteoglycan is also expressed strongly by natural collagen, and is an important component of the chondron, which protects chondrocytes in this tissue. Black inclusions are fibers of the scaffold

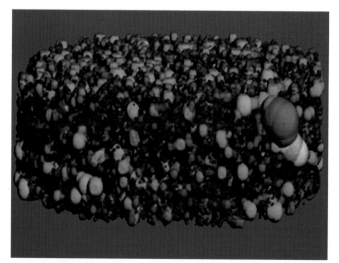

**Fig. 6.15:** MicroCT 3D reconstruction of pore spaces in a typical calcium phosphate scaffold, the large void (shown in red) is approximately 0.8 μm in diameter

hydrophobic surfaces in the culture tray, however, the cells can develop as clusters in suspension. This process avoids the introduction of exogenous factors in the cell development, and allows us to evaluate the influence of the serum medium, and community effects within the clusters.

## Characterization

Model engineered tissues are characterized using a range of techniques, including histology and immunocytochemistry, biochemical analysis of matrix, electron microscopy and MicroCT **(Fig. 6.17)**.

Histology allows us to examine and compare the distribution of a range of indicator matrix components in natural and engineered cartilage, for example:

- Various types of collagen (our interest is principally in types I, II, VI and X)
- Glucosaminoglycans and mineral deposition, important for engineering bone
- Surface enzymes, such as alkaline phosphotase, which is strongly expressed by osteocytes and hypertrophic chondrocytes
- Cell surface receptors, e.g. CD44, the expression of which is a measure of the cells continuing utility for clinical treatments.

Quantitative biochemical analysis allows us to evaluate absolute amounts of glycosaminoglycans, and real time PCR techniques permit us to examine levels of expression for matrix components such as aggrican, collagen I and II.

MicroCT (microcomputed tomography) is a useful technique for measuring pore sizes and permeability of solid supports for bone.

# Stem Cells in Gene Therapy

## DEFINITION

Genes, which are carried on chromosomes, are the basic physical and functional units of heredity. Genes are specific sequences of bases that encode instructions on how to make proteins. Although genes get a lot of attention, it's the proteins that perform most life functions and even make up the majority of cellular structures. When genes are altered so that the encoded proteins are unable to carry out their normal functions, genetic disorders can result.

Gene therapy is the insertion of genes into an individual's cells and tissues to treat a disease, and hereditary diseases in which a defective mutant allele is replaced with a functional one.

## PRINCIPLES AND PROMISE OF GENE THERAPY

Gene therapy is a relatively recent, and still highly experimental, approach to treating human disease. While traditional drug therapies involve the administration of chemicals that have been manufactured outside the body, gene therapy takes a very different approach: directing a patient's own cells to produce and deliver a therapeutic agent. The instructions for this are contained in the therapeutic transgene (the new genetic material introduced into the patient). Gene therapy uses genetic engineering-the introduction or elimination of specific genes by using molecular biology techniques to physically manipulate genetic material-to-alter or supplement the function of an abnormal gene by providing a copy of a normal gene, to directly repair such a gene, or to provide a gene that adds new functions or regulates the activity of other genes.

Clinical efforts to apply genetic engineering technology to the treatment of human diseases date back to 1989.

Initially, gene therapy clinical trials focused on cancer, infectious diseases, or disorders in which only a single gene is abnormal, such as cystic fibrosis. Increasingly, however, efforts are being directed toward complex, chronic diseases that involve more than one gene. Prominent examples include heart disease, inadequate blood flow to the limbs, arthritis, and Alzheimer's disease. The potential success of gene therapy technology depends not only on the delivery of the therapeutic transgene into the appropriate human target cells, but also on the ability of the gene to function properly in the cell. Both requirements pose considerable technical challenges.

## TYPES OF GENE THERAPY

Gene therapy researchers have employed two major strategies for delivering therapeutic transgenes into human recipients **(Fig. 7.1)**.

### Direct Delivery

The first is to "directly" infuse the gene into a person. Viruses that have been altered to prevent them from causing disease are often used as the vehicle for delivering the gene into certain human cell types, in much the same way as ordinary viruses infect cells. This delivery method is fairly imprecise and limited to the specific types of human cells that the viral vehicle can infect. For example, some viruses commonly used as gene-delivery vehicles, can only infect cells that are actively dividing. This limits their usefulness in treating diseases of the heart or brain, because these organs are largely composed of non dividing cells. Nonviral vehicles for directly delivering genes into cells are also being explored, including the use of plain DNA and DNA wrapped in a coat of fatty molecules known as liposomes.

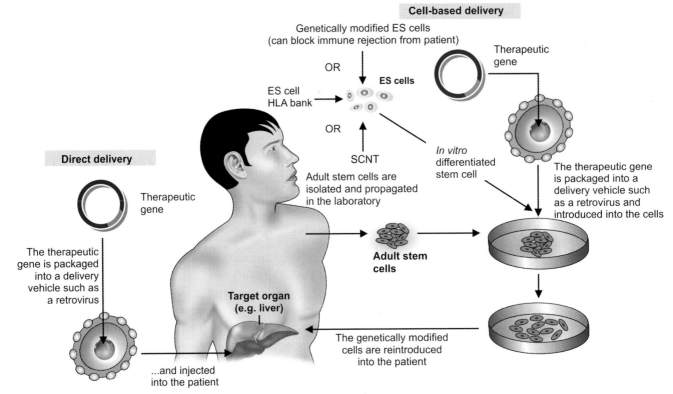

**Fig. 7.1:** Strategies for delivering therapeutic transgenes into patients

## Cell Based Delivery

The second strategy involves the use of living cells to deliver therapeutic transgenes into the body. In this method, the delivery cells often a type of stem cell, a lymphocyte, or a fibroblast-are removed from the body, and the therapeutic transgene is introduced into them via the same vehicles used in the previously described direct-gene-transfer method. While still in the laboratory, the genetically modified cells are tested and then allowed to grow and multiply and, finally, are infused back into the patient **(Fig. 7.2)**.

Gene therapy using genetically modified cells offers several unique advantages over direct gene transfer into the body and over cell therapy, which involves administration of cells that have not been genetically modified. First, the addition of the therapeutic transgene to the delivery cells takes place outside the patient, which allows researchers an important measure of control because they can select and work only with those cells that both contain the transgene and produce the therapeutic agent in sufficient quantity. Second, investigators can genetically engineer, or "program", the cells level and rate of production of the therapeutic agent. Cells can be programmed to steadily churn

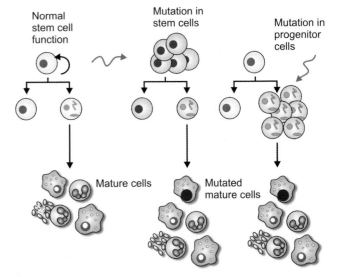

**Fig. 7.2:** Cell-based delivery

out a given amount of the therapeutic product. In some cases, it is desirable to program the cells to make large amounts of the therapeutic agent so that the chances that sufficient quantities are secreted and reach the diseased tissue in the patient are high. In other cases, it may be desirable to program the cells to produce the therapeutic agent in a regulated fashion. In this case, the therapeutic transgene would be active only in response to certain signals, such as drugs administered to the patient to turn the therapeutic transgene on and off.

Researchers may use one of several approaches for correcting faulty genes:

- A normal gene may be inserted into a nonspecific location within the genome to replace a nonfunctional gene. This approach is most common
- An abnormal gene could be swapped for a normal gene through homologous recombination

- The abnormal gene could be repaired through selective reverse mutation, which returns the gene to its normal function
- The regulation (the degree to which a gene is turned on or off) of a particular gene could be altered.

## VECTORS IN GENE THERAPY

In most gene therapy studies, a "normal" gene is inserted into the genome to replace an "abnormal", disease-causing gene. A carrier molecule called a vector must be used to deliver the therapeutic gene to the patient's target cells. Currently, the most common vector is a virus that has been genetically altered to carry normal human DNA. Viruses have evolved a way of

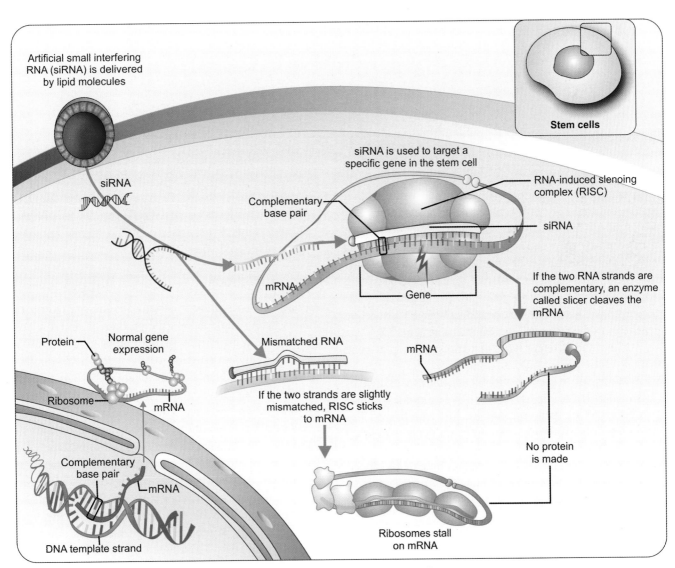

**Fig. 7.3:** RNA virus to modify stem cells

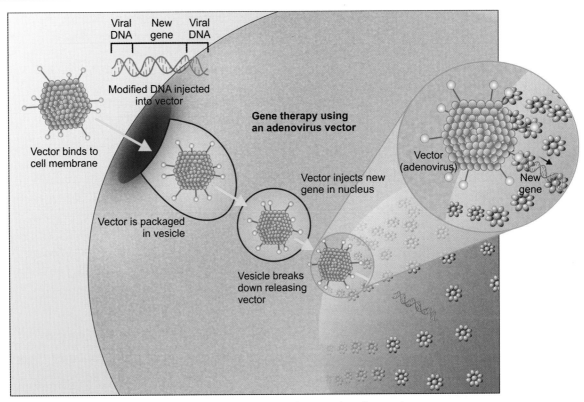

**Fig. 7.4:** Gene therapy using an adenovirus vector

encapsulating and delivering their genes to human cells in a pathogenic manner. Scientists have tried to take advantage of this capability and manipulate the virus genome to remove disease-causing genes and insert therapeutic genes. Target cells such as the patient's liver or lung cells are infected with the viral vector. The vector then unloads its genetic material containing the therapeutic human gene into the target cell. The generation of a functional protein product from the therapeutic gene restores the target cell to a normal state **(Fig. 7.3)**.

Some of the different types of viruses are used as gene therapy vectors **(Fig. 7.4)**:

- *Retroviruses:* A class of viruses that can create double-stranded DNA copies of their RNA genomes. These copies of its genome can be integrated into the chromosomes of host cells. Human immunodeficiency virus (HIV) is a retrovirus.
- *Adenoviruses:* A class of viruses with double-stranded DNA genomes that cause respiratory, intestinal, and eye infections in humans. The virus that causes the common cold is an adenovirus.
- *Adeno-associated viruses:* A class of small, single-stranded DNA viruses that can insert their genetic material at a specific site on chromosome.

- *Herpes simplex viruses:* A class of double-stranded DNA viruses that infect a particular cell type, neurons. Herpes simplex virus Type 1 is a common human pathogen that causes cold sores.

## Nonviral Methods

Nonviral methods present certain advantages over viral methods, with simple large scale production and low host immunogenicity being just two. Previously, low levels of transfection and expression of the gene held nonviral methods at a disadvantage; however, recent advances in vector technology have yielded molecules and techniques with transfection efficiencies similar to those of viruses.

- *Naked DNA:* This is the simplest method of nonviral transfection. Clinical trials carried out of intramuscular injection of a naked DNA plasmid have occurred with some success; however, the expression has been very low in comparison to other methods of transfection. In addition to trials with plasmids, there have been trials with naked PCR product, which have had similar or greater success. This success, however, does not compare to that of the other methods, leading to research into more efficient methods for delivery of the naked DNA such as electroporation and the use of a gun, which shoots DNA coated gold particles into the cell using high pressure gas.

- *Oligonucleotides:* The use of synthetic oligonucleotides in gene therapy is to inactivate the genes involved in the disease process. There are several methods by which this is achieved. One strategy uses antigen specific to the target gene to disrupt the transcription of the faulty gene. Another uses small molecules of RNA called siRNA to signal the cell to cleave specific unique sequences in the mRNA transcript of the faulty gene, disrupting translation of the faulty mRNA, and therefore expression of the gene. A further strategy uses double-stranded oligodeoxynucleotides as a decoy for the transcription factors that are required to activate the transcription of the target gene. The transcription factors bind to the decoys instead of the promoter of the faulty gene, which reduces the transcription of the target gene, lowering expression. Additionally, single-stranded DNA oligonucleotides have been used to direct a single base change within a mutant gene. The oligonucleotide is designed to anneal with complementarity to the target gene with the exception of a central base, the target base, which serves as the template base for repair. This technique is referred to as oligonucleotide mediated gene repair, targeted gene repair, or targeted nucleotide alteration.

- *Lipoplexes and polyplexes:* To improve the delivery of the new DNA into the cell, the DNA must be protected from damage and its entry into the cell must be facilitated. To this end new molecule, lipoplexes and polyplexes have been created that have the ability to protect the DNA from undesirable degradation during the transfection process. Plasmid DNA can be covered with lipids in an organized structure like a micelle or a liposome. When the organized structure is complexed with DNA it is called a lipoplex. There are three types of lipids, anionic (negatively charged), neutral, or cationic (positively charged). Initially, anionic and neutral lipids were used for the construction of lipoplexes for synthetic vectors. However, in spite of the facts that there is little toxicity associated with them, that they are compatible with body fluids and that there was a possibility of adapting them to be tissue specific; they are complicated and time consuming to produce therefore, attention was turned to the cationic versions. The most common use of lipoplexes has been in gene transfer into cancer cells, where the supplied genes have activated tumor

suppressor control genes in the cell and decrease the activity of oncogenes. Recent studies have shown lipoplexes to be useful in transfecting respiratory epithelial cells, so they may be used for treatment of genetic respiratory diseases such as cystic fibrosis. Complexes of polymers with DNA are called polyplexes. Most polyplexes consist of cationic polymers and their production is regulated by ionic interactions. One large difference between the methods of action of polyplexes and lipoplexes is that polyplexes cannot release their DNA load into the cytoplasm, so to this end, co-transfection with endosomelytic agents (to lyse the endosome that is made during endocytosis, the process by which the polyplex enters the cell) such as inactivated adenovirus must occur. However, this isn't always the case; polymers such as polyethylenimine have their own method of endosome disruption as does chitosan and trimethylchitosan.

Therapeutic DNA also can get inside target cells by chemically linking the DNA to a molecule that will bind to special cell receptors. Once bound to these receptors, the therapeutic DNA constructs are engulfed by the cell membrane and passed into the interior of the target cell. This delivery system tends to be less effective than other options.

## LIMITATIONS OF GENE THERAPY

- *Short-lived nature of gene therapy*: Before gene therapy can become a permanent cure for any condition, the therapeutic DNA introduced into target cells must remain functional and the cells containing the therapeutic DNA must be long-lived and stable. Problems with integrating therapeutic DNA into the genome and the rapidly dividing nature of many cells prevent gene therapy from achieving any long-term benefits. Patients will have to undergo multiple rounds of gene therapy.

- *Immune response:* Anytime a foreign object is introduced into human tissues, the immune system is designed to attack the invader. The risk of stimulating the immune system in a way that reduces gene therapy effectiveness is always a potential risk. Furthermore, the immune system's enhanced response to invaders, it has seen before, makes it difficult for gene therapy to be repeated in patients.

- *Problems with viral vectors:* Viruses, while the carrier of choice in most gene therapy studies, present a variety of potential problems to the patient-toxicity, immune and inflammatory responses, and gene control and targeting issues. In addition, there is always the fear that the viral vector, once inside the patient, may recover its ability to cause disease.

- *Multigene disorders:* Conditions or disorders that arise from mutations in a single gene are the best candidates for gene therapy. Unfortunately, some of the most commonly occurring disorders, such as heart disease, high blood pressure, Alzheimer,s disease, arthritis, and diabetes, are caused by the combined effects of variations in many genes. Multigene or multifactorial disorders such as these would be especially difficult to treat effectively using gene therapy.

## STEM CELLS IN GENE THERAPY

The intriguing biology of stem cells and their vast clinical potential is emerging rapidly for gene therapy. Bone marrow stem cells, including the pluripotent hematopoietic stem cells (HSCs), mesenchymal stem cells (MSCs) and possibly the multipotent adherent progenitor cells (MAPCs), are being considered as potential targets for cell and gene therapy-based approaches against a variety of different diseases **(Fig. 7.5)**.

The bone marrow (BM) is often used as a provider of stem cells for gene therapy approaches. The BM is composed of both non-adherent hematopoietic and adherent stromal cell compartments. Both the HSCs and the MSCs can self-renewal by proliferation and maintain their stem cell phenotype. The HSCs give rise to all different blood cell lineages, such as the myeloid and lymphoid cell lineages, and MSCs give rise to the stromal cells, which belong to the osteogenic, chondrogenic, adipogenic, myogenic and fibroblastic lineages. A more primitive adherent stem cell has recently been identified. This multipotent adult progenitor cell (MAPC) population can differentiate into MSCs, endothelial, epithelial and even hematopoietic cells. BM stem cells, including the pluripotent HSCs, MSCs and possibly the primitive MAPCs, are being considered as potential targets for cell and gene therapy-based approaches against a variety of different diseases. Although the use of stem cells may not overcome the usefulness of traditional medicines, gene therapy strategies involving stem cells in conjunction with the available drug regimens may help in better treatment options of otherwise incurable diseases.

Since the advent of gene therapy research, hematopoietic stem cells, have been a delivery-cell of choice for several reasons.

- First, although small in number, they are readily removed from the body via the circulating blood or bone marrow of adults or the umbilical cord blood of newborn infants.
- In addition, they are easily identified and manipulated in the laboratory and can be returned to patients relatively easily by injection.
- The ability of hematopoietic stem cells to give rise to many different types of blood cells means that once the engineered stem cells differentiate, the therapeutic transgene will reside in cells such as T and B lymphocytes, natural killer cells, monocytes, macrophages, granulocytes, eosinophils, basophils, and megakaryocytes.
- The clinical applications of hematopoietic stem cell-based gene therapies are thus also diverse, extending to organ transplantation, blood and bone marrow disorders, and immune system disorders.
- In addition, hematopoietic stem cells "home", or migrate, to a number of different spots in the body-primarily the bone marrow, but also the liver, spleen, and lymph nodes. These may be strategic locations for localized delivery of therapeutic agents for disorders unrelated to the blood system, such as liver diseases and metabolic disorders such as Gaucher's disease

Genetically manipulated MSCs may have direct applications to impact diseases in a variety of cell types in elaborate microenvironments and in different tissues *in situ*. The ability to genetically modify MSCs provides a means for durable expression of therapeutic genes for the lifetime of the patient for a wide range of diseases. MSCs can be engineered to secrete a variety of different proteins *in vitro* and *in vivo* that could potentially treat a variety of serum protein deficiencies and other genetic or acquired diseases, including bone, cartilage and BM disorders, or even cancer.

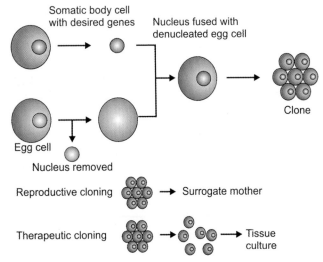

Fig. 7.5: Somatic body cell with desire genes

# Cancer Stem Cells

## DEFINITION

Cancer stem cells can be defined as cells in the tumor growth with a tumor initiating potential.

Compared to normal stem cells, the cancer stem cells are believed to have no control on the cell numbers. Cancer stem cells form very small numbers in whole tumor growth and they are said to be responsible for the growth of the tumor cells. It has been well-known that in order to induce a tumor in an animal model, hundreds of thousands of cancer cells need to be injected. This has been explained to be due to limitations in the assay to support tumor growth, or due to tumor formation deficiency. With the recent concept of the cancer stem cells, it may be explained that higher numbers of cancer cells are needed to maximize the probability of injecting cancer stem cells in animal model. At present, the shrinkage in the size of a tumor is considered as a response to the treatment. However, tumor often shrinks in response to the treatment only to recur again. This may be explained by cancer stem cells that the treatment targeting the cancer cells may not be able to target the cancer stem cells **(Figs 8.1 to 8.7)**.

A fundamental problem in the cancer is the identification of the cell type capable of sustaining the neoplastic growth. There is evidence that the majority of the cancers are clones and that the cancer cells represent the progeny of one cell, however, it is not clear which cells possess the tumor-initiating cell (TIC) function (cancer stem cells) and how to recognize them. Though the idea of cancer stem cells is considered as a new concept in science, it was thought almost 35 years back in 1971 when they were called as leukemic stem cells. A small subset of cancer cells capable of extensive proliferation in leukemia and multiple myeloma were found and named as leukemic stem cells (LSCs).

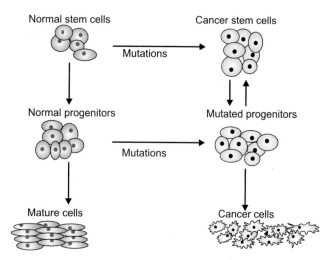

**Fig. 8.1:** A simplified model of suggested hypothesis about origin of the cancer stem cells

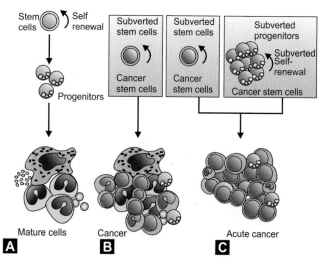

**Figs 8.2A to C:** Sources of cancer stem cells

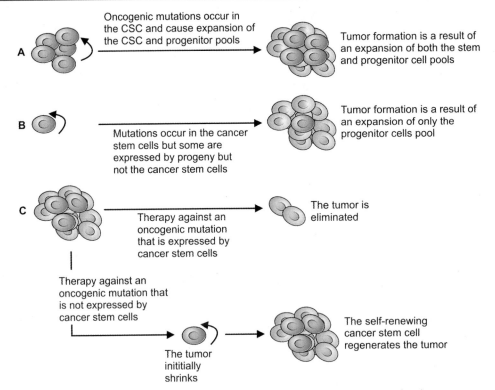

**Fig. 8.3:** Oncogenic mutation could affect either cancer stem cells or nontumorigenic progeny

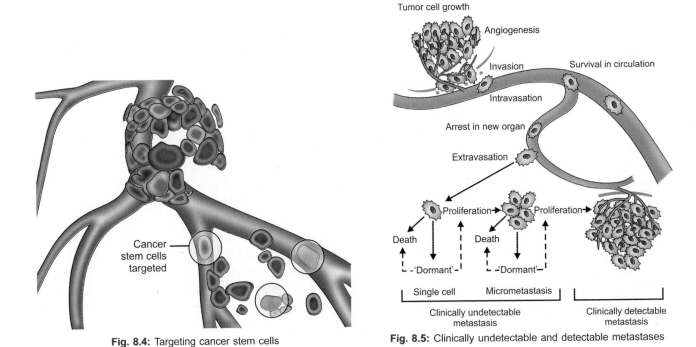

**Fig. 8.4:** Targeting cancer stem cells

**Fig. 8.5:** Clinically undetectable and detectable metastases

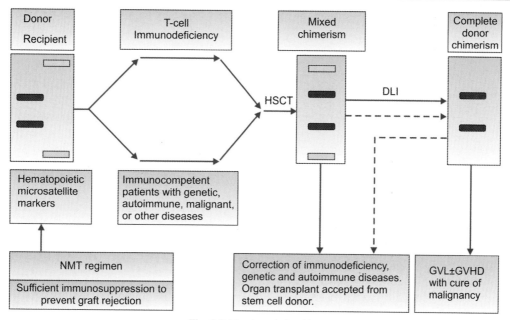

**Fig. 8.6:** Treatment algorithm

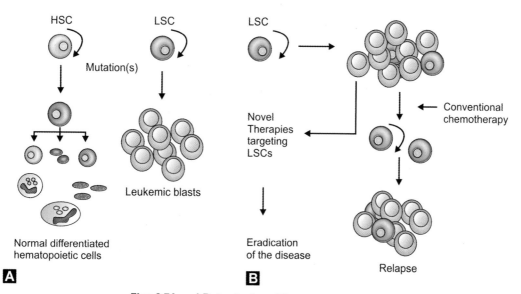

**Figs 8.7A and B:** Implication of the cancer stem cells

Two possibilities were proposed:
1. Either all leukemia cells had a low probability of proliferation and therefore all leukemia cells behave as LSC, or only a small subset was clonogenic.
2. The later theory was favored by Dick and colleagues who were able to separate the LSC as CD34 + CD38 – from patients' samples. Despite being small in numbers (0.2%), these were the only cells capable to transfer acute myeloid leukemia from patients to NOD-SCID (non-obese diabetic severe combined immunodeficiency) mice.

Recently, the cancer stem cells were also shown in the solid tumors such as breast cancer and brain tumors. The cancer stem cells have been shown to have not only self-renewal capability but also generating wide spectrum of progeny, like normal stem cells. In pediatric brain tumors, including medulloblastomas and gliomas, a subset of cells, called neurospheres, have been shown to have self-renewal capability. In conditions to promote differentiation, these neurospheres gave rise to neurons and glia, in proportion that reflect the amount in the tumor **(Figs 8.8 and 8.9)**.

### Targeting Leukemia Stem Cells

a. At present, treatment for leukemia uses chemo-therapeutic agents that target all leukemia cells (gray), based on properties such as their increased proliferation and entry into the cell cycle. However, it is likely that this approach spares the population of leukemia stem cell (LSCs; green), which are responsible for the continued growth and propagation of the tumor. In many instances, this leads to recurrence of the disease **(Fig. 8.10)**.

b. A greater understanding of LSC biology will allow us to design therapeutic agents that specifically target the LSC populations. Such therapies used alone, or in combination with conventional chemotherapeutic agents that reduce tumor burden, should lead to tumor involution or disease remission, respectively. Both of these approaches could improve both initial response rates and overall survival, through a decrease in the relapse of disease **(Figs 8.11 and 8.12)**.

## ORIGIN OF CANCER STEM CELLS

The cancer stem cells may be able to answer some of the questions related to a cancer growth, however origin of the cancer stem cells is yet to be defined. To recognize the origin of the cancer stem cells, two important factors need to be considered:
1. A number of mutations are required for a cell to be cancerous.
2. A stem cell needs to overcome any genetic constraints on both self-renewal and proliferation capabilities.

It is unlikely that all the mutations could occur in the life span of a progenitor/mature cell. Therefore, cancer stem cells should be derived from either the self-renewing normal stem cells or from the progenitor cells that have acquired the ability of self-renewal due to mutations. The hypothesis that cancer stem cells are derived from normal stem cells rather than more committed progenitor cells have been addressed in the cases of AML where leukemia initiating cells (LICs) from various subtypes of AML with different stages of differentiation have been shown to share the same

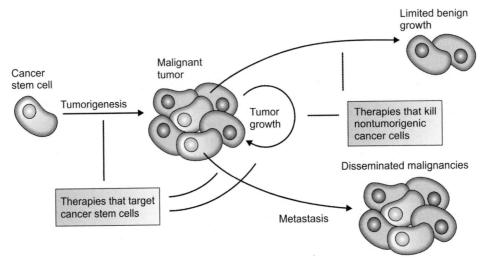

**Fig. 8.8:** Therapeutic implications of cancer stem cells

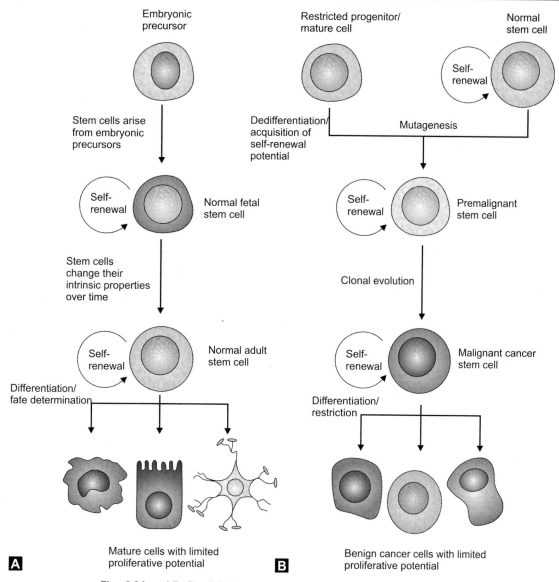

**Figs 8.9A and B:** Parallels between normal stem cells and cancer stem cells

cell-surface markers with normal hematopoietic stem cells. However, some of the studies have suggested that cancer stem cells can be derived from the normal stem cells, as well as from the committed short-lived progenitors, giving rise to the tumors with comparable latencies, phenotypes and gene expression profiles.

In the solid tumors, lack of the markers to characterize the tumor initiating cells (TICs) in the tumors has made it difficult to study the origins of the cancer stem cells, however, there have been identification of cell-surface markers in the lung, brain and prostate which may allow the separation of the stem or progenitor cells with the tumor initiating function **(Figs 8.13 and 8.14)**.

## CANCER STEM CELL PATHWAY

A normal stem cell may be transformed into a cancer stem cell through disregulation of the proliferation and differentiation pathways controlling it. Scientists working on cancer stem cells hope to design new drugs targeting these cellular mechanisms. The first findings in this area were made using hematopoietic stem cells (HSCs) and their transformed counterparts in leukemia, the disease whose stem cell origin is most strongly established. However, these pathways appear to be shared by stem cells of all organs **(Figs 8.15 and 8.16)**.

- *Bmi* - 1: The polycomb group transcriptional repressor Bmi-1 was discovered as a common oncogene activated

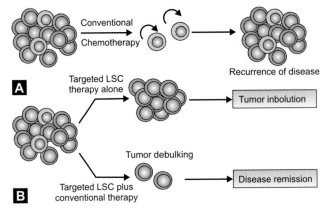

**Figs 8.10A and B:** Leukemia stem cells

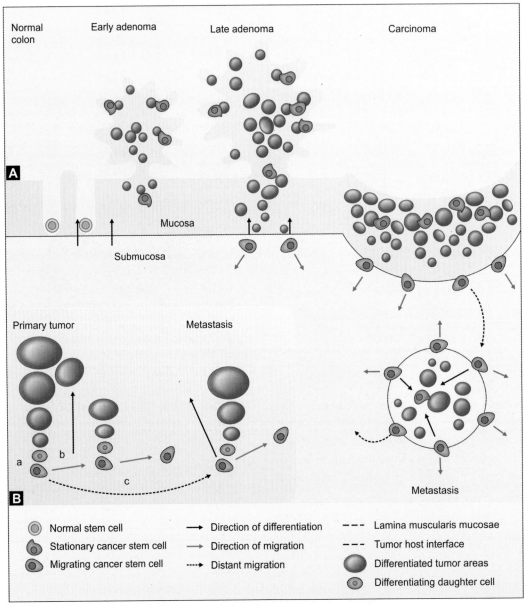

**Figs 8.11A and B:** Migrating cancer stem cell concept

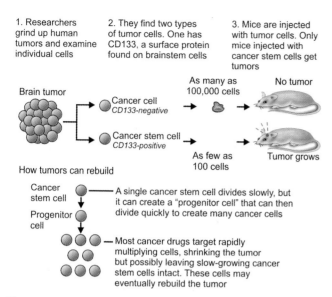

1. Researchers grind up human tumors and examine individual cells

2. They find two types of tumor cells. One has CD133, a surface protein found on brainstem cells

3. Mice are injected with tumor cells. Only mice injected with cancer stem cells get tumors

Brain tumor

Cancer cell *CD133-negative* → As many as 100,000 cells → No tumor

Cancer stem cell *CD133-positive* → As few as 100 cells → Tumor grows

How tumors can rebuild

Cancer stem cell → Progenitor cell → A single cancer stem cell divides slowly, but it can create a "progenitor cell" that can then divide quickly to create many cancer cells

Most cancer drugs target rapidly multiplying cells, shrinking the tumor but possibly leaving slow-growing cancer stem cells intact. These cells may eventually rebuild the tumor

**Fig. 8.12:** Which cells really cause cancer? Researchers in Toronto have shown that human brain tumors originate from cancer stem cells, and that these stem cells fuel and maintain growth of the tumors

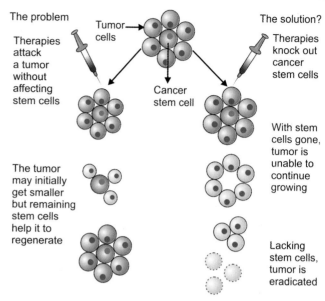

The problem — Therapies attack a tumor without affecting stem cells

Tumor cells

Cancer stem cell

The solution? — Therapies knock out cancer stem cells

With stem cells gone, tumor is unable to continue growing

The tumor may initially get smaller but remaining stem cells help it to regenerate

Lacking stem cells, tumor is eradicated

**Fig. 8.14:** The cancer stem cell theory. A very small percentage of cells in a tumor may be stem cells, the ones that make it so deadly. So to knock out cancer permanently, a therapy would have to attack these as well as regular tumor cells

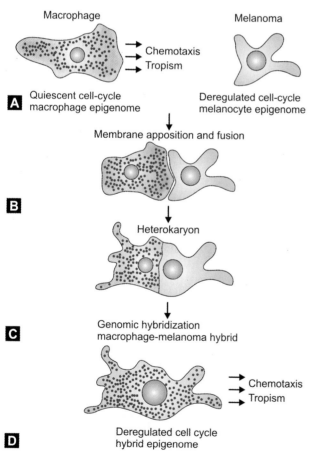

Macrophage — Chemotaxis — Tropism

Melanoma

**A** Quiescent cell-cycle macrophage epigenome

Deregulated cell-cycle melanocyte epigenome

Membrane apposition and fusion

**B**

Heterokaryon

**C**

Genomic hybridization macrophage-melanoma hybrid

**D** Deregulated cell cycle hybrid epigenome — Chemotaxis — Tropism

**Figs 8.13A to D:** A melanoma cell with a macrophage

in lymphoma and later shown to specifically regulate HSCs. The role of Bmi-1 has also been illustrated in neural stem cells. The pathway appears to be active in cancer stem cells of pediatric brain tumors.

- *Notch*: The notch pathway has been known to developmental biologists for decades. Its role in control of stem cell proliferation has now been demonstrated for several cell types including hematopoietic, neural and mammary stem cells. Components of the notch pathway have been proposed to act as oncogenes in mammary and other tumors.

- *Sonic hedgehog and Wnt*: These developmental pathways are also strongly implicated as stem cell regulators. Both Sonic hedgehog (SHH) and Wnt pathways are commonly hyperactivated in tumors and are required to sustain tumor growth. However, the Gli transcription factors that are regulated by SHH take their name from gliomas, where they are commonly expressed at high levels. A degree of crosstalk exists between the two pathways and their activation commonly goes hand-in-hand. This is a trend rather than a rule. For instance, in colon cancer hedgehog signaling appears to antagonize Wnt.

## IMPLICATIONS FOR CANCER TREATMENT

At present, the cancer treatment is targeted at its proliferation potential and its ability to metastasize, and hence the majority of treatments are targeted at rapidly dividing

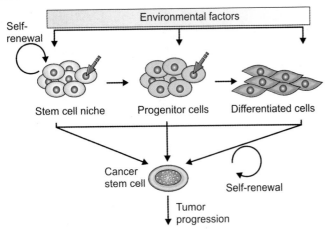

**Fig. 8.15:** Mutations in stem cells might give rise to cancer stem cells

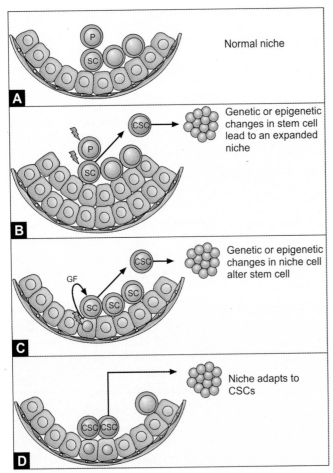

**Figs 8.16A to D:** Reciprocal interactions between the cancer stem cell and its microenvironment

cells and at molecular targets that represent the bulk of the tumor. This may explain the failure of treatments to eradicate the disease or the recurrence of the cancer. Although current treatments can shrink the size of the tumor, these effects are transient and usually do not improve patient's survival outcomes. For tumors in which the cancer stem cells play role, three possibilities exist.

- First, the mutation of normal stem cells or progenitor cells into cancer stem cells can lead to the development of the primary tumor.
- Second, during chemotherapy, most of the primary tumor cells may be destroyed but if cancer stem cells are not eradicated, they become refractory cancer stem cells and may lead to recurrence of tumor.
- Third, the cancer stem cells may emigrate to distal sites from the primary tumor and cause metastasis.

Theoretically, identification of the cancer stem cells may allow the development of treatment modalities that target the cancer stem cells rather than rapidly dividing cells in the cancer. This may cure the cancer as the remaining cells in the cancer growth have limited proliferative capability. If cytotoxic agents spare TICs, the disease is more likely to relapse. The TICs have been shown to have different sensitivity to different chemotherapeutic agents such as TICs in leukemia are less sensitive to daunorubicin and cytarabine. Although the idea of the therapies focused on the cancer stem cells may look exciting, targeting the cancer stem cells may not be easy **(Table 8.1 and Fig. 8.17)**.

The cancer stem cells are relatively quiescent compared to other cancer cells and do not appear to have the hyperproliferation signals activated such as tyrosine kinase. These make the cancer stem cells resistant to the toxicity of the anticancer drugs, which traditionally target the rapidly dividing cells. In addition, the tumor suppressor gene *PTEN* [106], polycomb gene Bmi1 and the signal transduction pathways such as the Sonic Hedgehog (Shh), Notch and Wnt that are crucial for normal stem cell regulation, have been shown to be deregulated in the process of carcinogenesis. These deregulated signalling pathways and gene expressions may have impact on response to cancer therapy. One approach to target the cancer stem cells may be the identification of the markers that are specific for the cancer stem cells compared to normal stem cells such as hematopoietic stem cells express Thy-1 and percent-kit whereas leukemic stem cells express IL-3 (interleukin-3) receptor α-chain.

Although the origin of the cancer stem cells is yet to be defined, the concept of the cancer stem cells may allow new treatment options in the possible cure of the cancer. However, further research is required to identify and separate the cancer stem cells in various cancers from normal stem cells and other cancer cells **(Fig. 8.18)**. Further work is also required to differentiate the genes and signalling pathways in the process of the carcinogenesis from cancer stem cells for development of new therapies, with the eventual goal of eliminating the residual disease and recurrence.

**TABLE 8.1:** Cancer surface markers with cancer types

| Cancer type | Cell surface markers | | | | | | | | | Reference |
| | CD133 | CD44 | CD24 | CD34 | CD38 | CD117 | Nanog | Oct-3/4 | Total % of tumor | |
|---|---|---|---|---|---|---|---|---|---|---|
| Brain tumors | + | | | | | | | | 0.3 to 25.1% | Singh et al 2003 |
| Prostate cancer | + | | | | | | | | | Lang et al 2008 |
| Colon cancer | + | | | | | | | | 0.002% | O'Brien et al 2007 |
| Lung cancer | + | | | | | | | | 5 to 30% | Eramo et al 2007 |
| Hepatic carcinoma | + | | | | | | | | | Suetsugu et al 2006 |
| Breast cancer | | + | – | | | | | | | A1-Hajj et al 2002 |
| Ovarian cancer | | + | | | | + | + | + | 0.20% | Zhang et al 2008 |
| Pancreatic cancer | | + | + | | | | | | 0.2 to 0.8% | Li et al 2007 |
| Head and neck squamous Cell carcinoma | | + | | | | | | | < 10% | Prince et al 2006 |
| Acute myeloid leukemia | | | | + | – | | | | | Bonnet and Dick, 1997 |

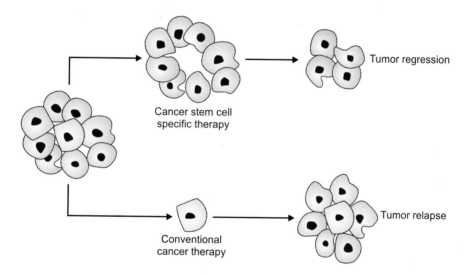

**Fig. 8.17:** The conventional therapies may shrink the size of the tumor; by contrast, if the therapies are directed against the cancer stem cells, they are more effective in eradicating the tumor

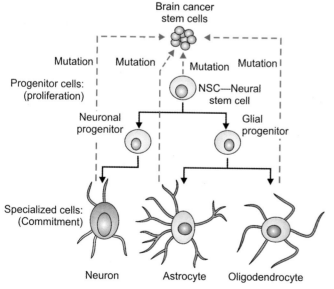

**Fig. 8.18:** Brain cancer stem cells and neural stem cells: After exploring the possible derivations of brain cancer stem cells, oncogenic mutations in adult neural cells and mutated neuronal stem cells have the experimental evidence supporting them as causes for the development of brain cancer stem cells. This diagram depicts what may be occurring when brain cancer stem cells form

# Stem Cells in Dental Tissue

## STEM CELLS IN TEETH

While stem cells can be found in most tissues of the body, they are usually buried deep, are few in number and are similar in appearance to surrounding cells. With the discovery of stem cells in teeth, an accessible and available source of stem cells has been identified. The tooth is nature's "safe" for these valuable stem cells, and there is an abundance of these cells in baby teeth, wisdom teeth and permanent teeth. The stem cells contained within teeth are capable of replicating themselves and can be readily recovered at the time of a planned dental procedure. Living stem cells found within extracted teeth were routinely discarded every day, but now, with the knowledge from recent medical research, gives you the opportunity to save these cells for future use in developing medical treatments for your family. Aside from being the most convenient stem cells to access, dental stem cells have significant medical benefits in the development of new medical therapies.

Using one's own stem cells for medical treatment means a much lower risk of rejection by the body and decreases the need for powerful drugs that weaken the immune system, both of which are negative but typical realities that come into play when tissues or cells from a donor are used to treat patients. Further, the stem cells from teeth have been observed in research studies to be among the most powerful stem cells in the human body. Stem cells from teeth replicate at a faster rate and for a longer period of time than do stem cells harvested from other tissues of the body. Stem cells in the human body age over time and their regenerative abilities slow down later in life. The earlier in life that a family's stem cells are secured, the more valuable they will be when they are needed most.

## TOOTH ELIGIBILITY CRITERIA—MOST PROLIFERATIVE STAGE

A healthy pulp contains viable stem cells. For a pulp to be considered healthy, the tooth must have:
*   An intact blood supply
*   Be free of infection, deep caries and other pathologies.
    Stem cells are not concentrated within any particular area of a healthy pulp, but are diffusely spread throughout the cellular zone adjacent to the nerve and blood vessels within the pulp. Specific criteria must be met in order for a tooth to be eligible for stem cell recovery. This can be broken down into three distinct tooth groups in which patients have the opportunity to recover their stem cells. It is best to recover stem cells when a patient is young and healthy and the stem cells are at their most proliferative. Stem cells can also be recovered from the permanent teeth of middle-aged individuals. Benefits are realized at this age when compared to current life-expectancy statistics, coupled with the almost certain need for their use in future regenerative therapies.

### Deciduous Teeth

The healthy pulps of deciduous teeth are a rich source of viable stem cells. Scientific data supports that stem cells isolated from healthy pulp of deciduous teeth are highly proliferative, even when the pulp is recovered in small quantities.

Certain factors will determine whether viable stem cells can be recovered from deciduous teeth:
*   The ideal deciduous tooth for stem cell recovery is a canine or incisor that has just started to loosen, has more than a third of the root structure left intact, and is not extracted for reasons such as infection or associations with pathology **(Figs 9.1A to C)**.

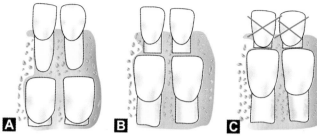

**Figs 9.1A to C:** Ideal candidates for stem cell recovery include deciduous teeth that still possess some root structure and a healthy pulp

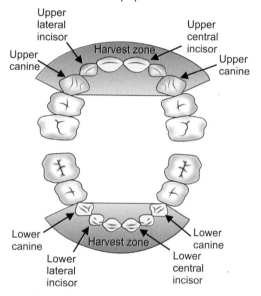

**Fig. 9.2:** The harvest zone for stem cells

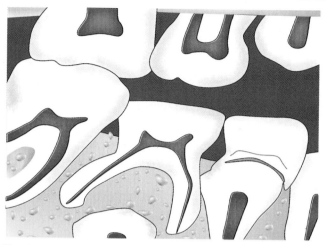

**Fig. 9.3:** Deciduous molars have an unpredictable amount of viable pulpal tissue at the time of exfoliation and are not always good candidates for stem cell recovery

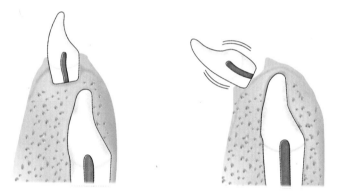

**Fig. 9.4:** Necrotic pulp

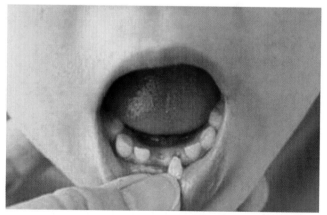

**Fig. 9.5:** Teeth that are "hanging on by a thread" are not candidates for stem cell recovery

- Supernumerary or mesodens are another ideal source for dental stem cells. In most cases when these teeth are removed, they still have a complete root, intact blood supply and healthy pulp.
- Harvest zone: The harvest zone for stem cells is from the deciduous canine to canine **(Fig. 9.2)**.
- Deciduous molars may have their pulp chambers obliterated by the erupting permanent bicuspids by the time they become loose. In most cases, the remaining pulpal tissue may not be adequate for dental stem cell recovery. Over-retained molars and molars extracted for orthodontic reasons may also be considered **(Fig. 9.3)**.
- The pulps of naturally exfoliated teeth or teeth that have fallen out on their own are most likely necrotic, as they have been separated from their blood supply. A patient bringing a tooth in hand to the office is not a good candidate for recovery **(Fig. 9.4)**.
- An excessively loose tooth or one that is "hanging on by a thread" is not a candidate for stem cell recovery. Even though the tooth is still attached to gingiva, the pulp most likely is necrotic **(Fig. 9.5)**.

## Wisdom Teeth

The healthy pulp from wisdom teeth is another excellent source for viable stem cells. Whole or sectioned portions of third molars containing healthy pulp can be recovered at the time of their removal. When an impacted third molar needs to be sectioned for removal, the pulp is often exposed.

- Developing third molars have a larger volume of pulpal tissue than teeth that are mature with their roots completely formed **(Fig. 9.6)**.
- It is best to recover these teeth during the developmental stage (between 16 and 20 years of age), when the stem cells are very active in the formation of the root and supporting root structures.
- Third molars with healthy pulp can also be recovered later in life and are always considered a source for viable stem cells.

## Permanent Teeth

All permanent teeth with healthy pulp are potential sources of stem cells.

- Bicuspids needing to be removed for orthodontic indications are an example of this.
- Permanent teeth to avoid include: Endodontically-treated or nonviable teeth, teeth with active infections, teeth with severe periodontal disease and excessive mobility, teeth with deep caries or large restorations, and teeth with sclerosing or calcified pulp chambers.
- Age is important. The stem cells from within the pulp become less proliferative as individuals age, so it is best to recover stems cells at the earliest opportunity **(Figs 9.7 and 9.8)**.

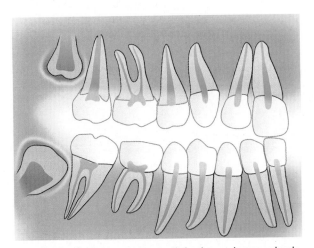

**Fig. 9.6:** Developing wisdom teeth having an increased pulp chamber

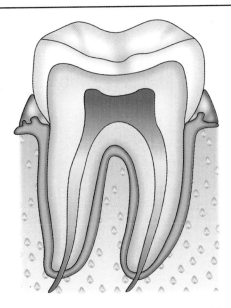

**Fig. 9.7:** Healthy pulp molar of 18-year-old

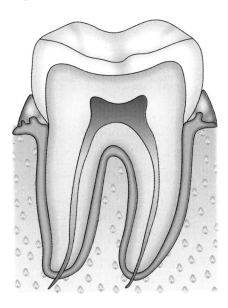

**Fig. 9.8:** Sclerosed pulp molar of 60-year-old

## STEM CELL RECOVERY

Stem cells are unique because they drive the natural healing process throughout life. Stem cells are different from other cells in the body because they regenerate and produce specialized cell types. They heal and restore skin, bones, cartilage, muscles, nerves and other tissues when injured **(Figs 9.9 and 9.10)**.

As a result, amazing new medical treatments are being developed to treat a range of diseases contemporary medicine currently deems difficult or impossible to treat. Among them are:

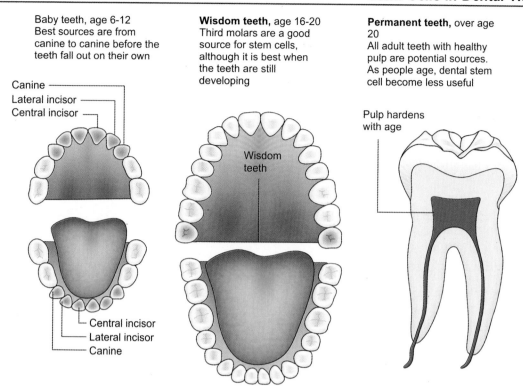

Baby teeth, age 6-12
Best sources are from canine to canine before the teeth fall out on their own

Canine
Lateral incisor
Central incisor

Central incisor
Lateral incisor
Canine

**Wisdom teeth,** age 16-20
Third molars are a good source for stem cells, although it is best when the teeth are still developing

Wisdom teeth

**Permanent teeth,** over age 20
All adult teeth with healthy pulp are potential sources. As people age, dental stem cell become less useful

Pulp hardens with age

**Fig. 9.9:** Recovering stem cells: companies collecting stem cells say it is best to recover them when patients are young, but they can be retrieved at any age if the teeth are healthy

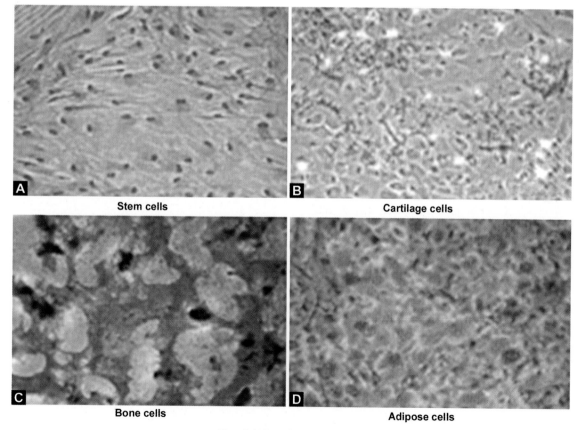

A — Stem cells

B — Cartilage cells

C — Bone cells

D — Adipose cells

**Figs 9.10A to D:** Types of cells

- Parkinson's disease
- Brain injuries
- Heart disease
- Diabetes
- Arthritis
- Muscular dystrophy
- Leukemia
- Crohn's disease
- Multiple sclerosis
- Periodontal disease
- Sports injuries
- Cosmetic and anti-aging applications.

## Advantages of Stem Cell Recovery and Cryopreservation from Teeth

*Accessible:* The stem cells contained within teeth are recovered at the time of a planned procedure; for example, Extraction of wisdom teeth, baby teeth or other healthy permanent teeth.

*Affordable and less invasive:* When compared with other methods of acquiring and preserving life-saving stem cells: Peripheral blood, bone marrow, cord blood, etc.

*Convenience:* The recovery of stem cells from teeth can be performed in the doctor's office anytime when a healthy tooth is being extracted.

*Ease of use:* The recovery of stem cells from teeth does not add any additional time on to a planned procedure.

## Dental Stem Cell Banking

### Why store dental stem cells?

Cell preservation technology makes it possible to save valuable stem cells for the day, possibly years in the future, when it may be needed. Rather than discarding these cells and hoping that another source will be available in the future, one can set their own cells aside, knowing that it can be obtained if and when they are needed.

Stem cell banking has existed for years. Many families have already preserved stem cells for their children, by banking umbilical cord blood. Now, with the discovery of stem cells in baby teeth and wisdom teeth, a second chance is available for those families who missed their opportunity to store cord blood, as well as a chance to add a new type of stem cells for those families who did.

Banking stem cells is simple. Instead of throwing away the tooth, the dentist will send it to the laboratory, where the tooth will be processed and the stem cells safely frozen. If ever needed, it can be obtained from the laboratory.

## The Process

Step 1: Tooth collection **(Fig. 9.11)**
Once the tooth is obtained from the child, it is placed in the collection box and delivered to the laboratory.

Step 2: Stem cell isolation **(Fig. 9.12)**
On receiving the tooth, all the cells are isolated. Then the current health and viability of these cells are analyzed.

Step 3: Tooth cell storage **(Fig. 9.13)**
Cryopreservation of the tooth cells is then done for future use. **(Fig. 9.14)**
The sample is then divided into four cryotubes and each part is stored in a separate location in our cryogenic system. This means that, in the unlikely event of a problem with one

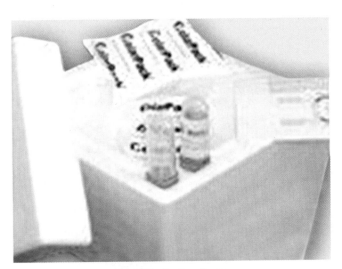
**Fig. 9.11:** Tooth collection

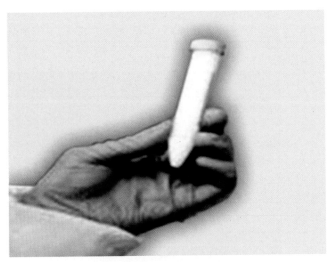
**Fig. 9.12:** Stem cell isolation

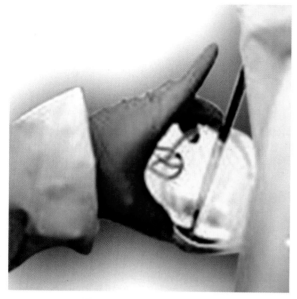

Fig. 9.13: Tooth cell storage

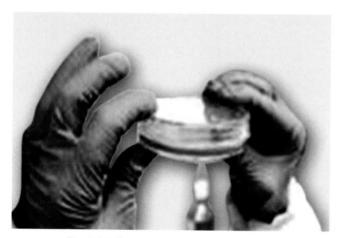

Fig. 9.14: Cryopreservation of the tooth cells

of the storage units, there will be another sample available for use. The cells are then preserved in liquid nitrogen vapor at a temperature of less than –150°C. This preserves the cells and maintains their potential potency.

The first 48 hours after the tooth is out of the mouth are critical. The tooth must be prepared, packaged and received at laboratory during this time to maximize a successful isolation.

## About Tooth Stem Cells

Stem cell therapy is emerging as a revolutionary new way to treat disease and injury, with wide-ranging medical benefits. It works by introducing stem cells into an area

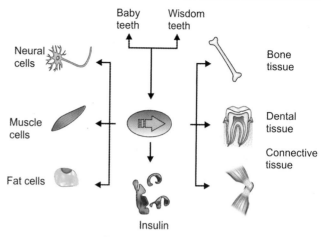

Fig. 9.15: Tooth stem cell

where the normal cells have lost their function due to disease or damage. The stem cells then replace or repair the damaged cells and restore normal function **(Fig. 9.15)**.

## Different Types of Tooth Stem Cells

1. *Adipocytes*: Adipocytes have successfully been used to repair damage to the heart muscle caused by severe heart attack. There is also preliminary data to indicate they can be used to treat cardiovascular disease, spine and orthopedic conditions, congestive heart failure, Crohn's disease, and can be used in plastic surgery.
2. *Chondrocytes and osteoblasts*: Chondrocytes and osteoblasts have successfully been used to grow bone and cartilage suitable for transplant. They have also been used to grow intact teeth in animals.
3. *Mesenchymal*: Mesenchymal stem cells have successfully been used to repair spinal cord injury and to restore feeling and movement in paralyzed human patients. Since they can form neuronal clusters, mesenchymal stem cells also have the potential to treat neuronal degenerative disorders such as Alzheimer's and Parkinson's diseases, cerebral palsy, as well as a host of other disorders. Mesenchymal stem cells have more therapeutic potential than any other type of adult stem cells.

## DENTAL PULP STEM CELLS

Although the regenerative capacity of the human dentin/pulp complex is not well-understood, it is known that, upon injury, reparative dentin is formed as a protective barrier for the pulp. Accordingly, one might anticipate that dental pulp contains the dentinogenic progenitors that are responsible for dentin repair. Previous work has shown that dental pulp contains proliferating cells that are analogous to bone cells, because they express osteogenic markers and respond to many growth factors for osteo/odontogenic differentiation. In addition, dental pulp cells are capable of forming mineral deposits with distinctive dentin-like crystalline structures. Recently, dental pulp stem cells (DPSCs) have been isolated from extracted human third molars.

Another mineralized tissue that has a great deal of similarity to bone is dentin. Although dentin is not turned over throughout life, as is bone, limited dentinal repair in the postnatal organism does occur. It was postulated that the ability for limited repair is maintained by a precursor population, associated with pulp tissue that has the ability to mature into odontoblasts. Clonogenic and highly proliferative cells have been derived from enzymatically disaggregated adult human dental pulp, which have been termed dental pulp stem cells (DPSCs) that form sporadic, but densely calcified nodules *in vitro*.

When DPSCs were transplanted with hydroxyapatite/tricalcium phosphate into immunocompromised mice, they generated a dentin-like structure with collagen fibers running perpendicular to the mineralizing surface as is found *in vivo*, and contained the dentin-enriched protein, dentin sialophosphoprotein. The newly formed dentin was lined with human odontoblasts like cells that extended long cellular processes into the mineralized matrix, and surrounded an interstitial tissue reminiscent of pulp *in vivo* with respect to the organization of the vasculature and connective tissue **(Figs 9.16 to 9.19)**. In contrast to BMSCs, DPSCs did not support the establishment of a hematopoietic marrow or adipocytes, elements that are also absent in dental pulp tissue *in vivo*. By immunophenotyping, the DSPCs are virtually identical to BMSCs, yet each population produces quite different mineralized matrices. To identify possible differences between these two populations, their gene expression profiles were characterized using a commercially available microarray.

## PERIODONTAL LIGAMENT STEM CELLS (Fig. 9.20)

The periodontal ligament (PDL) connects the cementum to alveolar bone, and functions primarily to support the tooth in the alveolar socket. A recent report identified stem cells in human PDL (PDLSCs) and found that PDLSCs implanted into nude mice generated cementum/PDL-like structures that resemble the native PDL as a thin layer of cementum that interfaced with dense collagen fibers, similar to Sharpey's fibers. After a three-week culture with an adipogenic-inductive cocktail, PDLSCs differentiated into oil red-o-positive, lipid-laden adipocytes. Upon four-week osteo/odontogenic inductions, alizarin-red-positive nodules formed in the PDLSC cultures, similar to MSCs and DPSCs. Thus, the PDLSCs have the potential for forming periodontal structures, including the cementum and PDL.

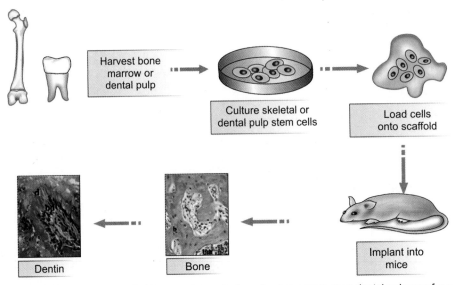

**Fig. 9.16:** Transplantation studies have shown that human stem cells from the bone marrow or dental pulp can form bone or dentin *in vivo*

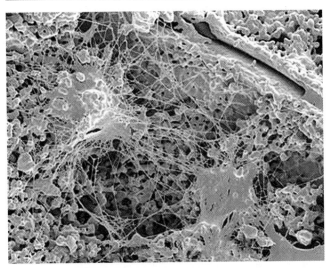

**Fig. 9.17:** Dental pulp stem cells grown for 8 days on a porous ceramic (calcium phosphate) scaffold with extensive formation of matrix proteins

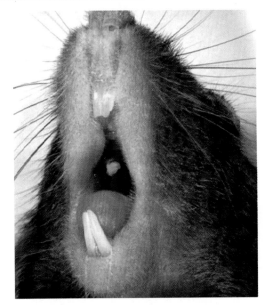

**Fig. 9.19:** Green glowing mouse tooth

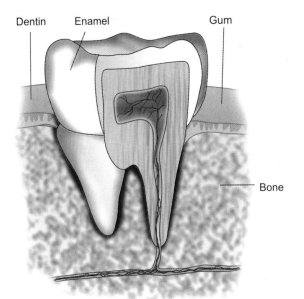

**Fig. 9.18:** Pulling stem cells from teeth: Research involving stem cells in teeth has exploded during the past four or five years and companies that will bank the cells in a deep-freeze have since begun operating. Company officials and their scientists say dental stem cells have the potential to treat a variety of diseases, including heart disease, leukemia and Parkinson. In the nearer future, dental stem cells could grow new teeth and jaw bone. Other scientists caution people against spending money to bank their stem cells

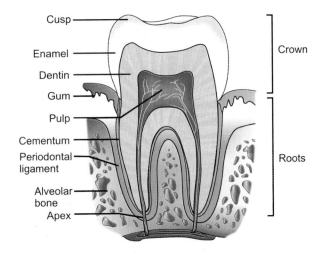

**Fig. 9.20:** Suppression of immune cells

## Gum Stem Cells

### Introduction

The periodontium is the area of specialized tissue surrounding the tooth and anchoring it to the underlying alveolar bone

**(Fig. 9.21)**. It is composed of four regions; the cementum, periodontal ligament (PDL), gingival (gums), and the alveolar bone. The cementum is a layer of mesenchymal tissue that surrounds the root of the tooth. Its main function is to serve as the site to which the PDL attaches. The other end of the PDL then attaches to the alveolar bone, therefore, anchoring the tooth in place. The PDL is composed of cells that have either fibroblastic or osteoblastic properties.

Periodontal disease is a bacterial infection that leads to tissue damage of the periodontium and is the major cause of tooth loss. The PDL goes through limited regeneration and repair if there is no therapeutic involvement. The current therapeutic methods are also somewhat ineffective in that

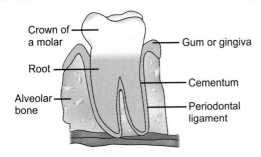

Fig. 9.21: Cross-section of a molar and the surrounding tissue

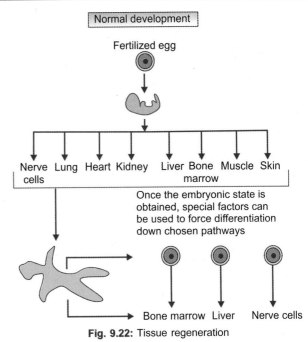

Fig. 9.22: Tissue regeneration

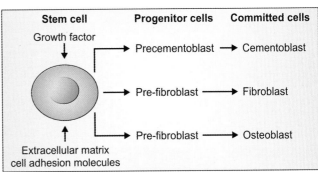

Fig. 9.23: Differentiation of adult mesenchymal stem cells and progenitor cells into PDL cells

they have variable efficacy as well as safety issues among other things. There are novel approaches to PDL regeneration that involve tissue engineering. It is in these new methods that the potential for the use of stem cells can be applied.

## Background

Stem cell is a term that refers to any number of cells that are able to self-renew and are not committed to being any one specific cell type. Adult stem cells are multipotent and can differentiate into any number of different cells, though this potential to differentiate is more limited than in embryonic stem cells. However, unlike embryonic stem cells there are fewer ethical and governmental restrictions when dealing with adult stem cells. Also, the use of adult stem cells can prove to be a more practical choice when dealing with tissue regeneration. Embryonic stem cells also have a high potential for tumorigenesis making them less desirable to use than the adult stem cells **(Fig. 9.22)**. To date, no studies have been done to assess the tumorigenic potential of PDLSCs.

Mesenchymal stem cells (MSCs) differentiate into different types of connective tissue such as muscle, endothelial cells, fibroblasts, osteoblasts, adipocytes and chondroblasts. Since, it is these types of cells that make up the tissue of the periodontium, it is determined that the PDL cells are derived from mesenchymal stem cells. The periodontal ligament stem cells (PDLSCs) are indeed a specialized MSCs **(Fig. 9.23)**.

Flow cytometry assays are often done in order to separate and identify certain cell populations. This is achieved by using a laser beam to separate cells based on the specific light-absorbing or fluorescing properties of these cells. The properties that are used to identify the specific populations of cells are cell surface markers that are unique to those populations. These markers are antigens that are expressed on certain cells and not others and can be identified using antibodies that are specific for those antigens. The flow cytometry method often used is Fluorescence-Activated Cell Sorting (FACS).

Generally, when stem cells differentiate into committed cells, they go through different phases of development. Before they can become fully differentiated cells, the stem cells go through an intermediate phase. At this point, the cells are somewhat differentiated and are considered progenitor cells. These progenitor cells must undergo further replications and differentiation before they reach the stage at which they are considered fully differentiated and committed cells. The PDLSC differentiate into three different cells in order to make up the tissues of the cementum, PDL, gingival and alveolar bone. These include cementoblasts, fibroblasts and osteoblasts.

## Identification and Location of the PDLSC

Scientists have believed for a couple of decades that there were progenitor cells located within the periodontal ligament that could differentiate into bone, cementum and extracellular matrix of the PDL. This is due to the observation of slow cycling time in populations of cells found in the PDL. However, it was not until 2004 that a group of scientists isolated these cells and were able to show that they were indeed stem cells. The PDLSC were isolated from the PDL of wisdom teeth and molars.

The stem cells required to form the types of tissues found in the periodontium, such as the cementum, ligament and bone are of mesenchymal origin. Also, the presence of all these varying cell types in the PDL led scientist to believe that they had a common origin which would be a progenitor stem cell. Therefore, markers for mesenchymal stem cells were used to isolate the stem cells found in the PDL. Progenitor cells were located in the paravascular regions of the PDL that originated from the spaces in the alveolar bone. These cells then differentiate and multiply and move to the different areas near the cementum and alveolar bone.

No specific cell markers are currently known in order to identify the exact location of these stem cells. However, STRO-1 was used to identify a general group of mesenchymal stem cells in the paravascular regions of the PDL. STRO-1 is a cell surface marker for mesenchymal stem cells but is not found in hematopoietic stem cells. However, the use of only STRO-1 is not sufficient to identify and locate PDLSCs. Therefore, other MSC surface markers, such as CD146 and CD44 were also used **(Table 9.1)**. The cell staining for these various markers confirmed that the PDLSCs were mainly located in the paravascular region of the PDL.

Two different cell morphologies were located in the paravascular region of the PDL. The first were cells that elongated nuclei and elongated cytoplasm and were typically found near the blood vessels of the PDL. These cells resemble endothelial cells and therefore could be the reason that studies vary in the number of PDL cells that are stem cells because they could in fact be endothelial cells. The second phenotype of cell seen in the paravascular region of the PDL that stained positive for MSC markers were round or oval shaped. They had prominent nuclei, very little cytoplasm and a great deal of hematoxylin staining. These second phenotypes of cells are more likely the stem cells whereas the first type could be cells that have already gone through differentiation.

## Properties of PDLSC

1. *Self-renewal*: PDL fibroblast cell populations show a capacity for self-renewal. This is one of the criteria that mark them as stem cells. This self-renewal is seen in the ability for the PDL to rapidly turnover. Though there is little regeneration of the periodontium when there is mechanical damage due to periodontitis, therefore, the self-renewal could be responsible for maintaining the PDL. This ability to self-renew was studied by using colony forming assays. It was found that when the PDL cells were plated at low densities they were able to form colonies successfully. Cells were also plated and used in transplantation into NOD/SCID mouse to show that they were able to regenerate tissue that had been damaged.

2. *Multipotency*: Another characteristic of PDLSCs is that they are able to differentiate into a number of different cells. Their potential to differentiate was studied by running colony forming assays using different induction methods. PDLSCs are able to form adipocytes, so adipogenesis was performed in a colony forming assay to determine the potential for the cells to differentiate into these types of cells. This was done by using a adipogenic medium and showed that there was indeed the formation of lipid rich vacuoles within the colonies. Similar colony forming assays

| Positive markers | Function |
| --- | --- |
| **TABLE 9.1:** Different positive marker.s of mesenchymal stem cells and their function ||
| **CD 105** | A component of the TGF beta receptor complex and is highly expressed on the surface of endothelial cells. It is important in angiogenesis. |
| **CD 146** | Belongs to the immunoglobin superfamily. It is a potential adhesion molecule in endothelial cells. |
| **CD 44** | Involved in cell-cell interactions as well as adhesion and migration of cells. |
| **Scleraxis** | A tendon specific transcription factor. PDLSCs express a higher level of scleraxis than other stem cells found in teeth, making them unique from other mesenchymal stem cells. |
| **CD 166** | A adhesion molecule that binds to CD. |
| **STRO-1** | An immunoglobulin antibody also used to detect stromal cells in human bone marrow. |

were done to study calcification potential. These colony forming assays supported the evidence of stem cells in the PDL because of the cell's ability to differentiate into different types of cells.

## Markers of PDLSCs

PDLSCs are a specialized mesenchymal stem cell (MSC). Therefore, they express markers that are similar to those used to identify MSCs. A specific antigen marker does not exist for MSCs or PDLSCs. Therefore, a combination of markers that are found on MSCs but not on hemopoietic stem cells must be used in order to identify the cells.

## Regulation of Differentiation

During development, it is believed that the tissue of the periodontium originates from the dental follicle. Once the periodontium is formed, the exact factors that regulate growth and differentiation are not well understood, yet. There have been several protein factors that have been identified to play a role in regulating the type of tissue that PDL cells can differentiate to. The growth factor FGF5, has been shown to induce the maintenance of the naïve state of the PDL cells and causes the cells to proliferate. The growth factor bone morphogenic protein-7 (BMP-7) induces the PDL cells to mineralize at the ends of the ligaments to connect the alveolar bone to the cementum. Growth differentiation factor-5 (GDF-5), induces the PDL to differentiate into a nonmineralized ligament that is bundled together to form the body of the ligament. Interestingly, there is evidence that differentiation is regulated differently in progenitor cells of the PDL when compared to the mature cells within the PDL. This knowledge is important if one attempts to induce a PDLSC to differentiate to a particular type of cell.

## Transplantation

A long-term goal for dentist would be to use tissue engineering techniques and PDLSCs to regenerate damaged areas within the oral cavity, in order to restore the original function and connection between the alveolar bone and the cementum in order to prevent tooth loss. PDLSCs show potential in having an important role in clinical use because they are able to differentiate into the different forms of tissue found within the periodontium. On top of that researchers have been able to identify, isolate and expand *ex vivo* PDLSC cells in mouse models. In these mouse models, PDLSC have been retrieved from PDL tissues that were isolated

from an extracted wisdom tooth. The PDL tissue were then treated and expanded to favor the proliferation of PDLSC. Then using techniques that created a favorable microenvironment and with the combination of hydroxyapatite/tricalcium phosphate (HA/TCP) to induce differentiation, these stem cells were injected subcutaneously at the site of damage within the oral cavity to immune deficient mice. The results of these experiments saw evidence for regeneration of the tissue within the periodontium, including the PDL ligament and gave great hope in having cell transplantation from donor to recipient one day **(Fig. 9.24)**. However, before such a treatment can be tested on humans, further research with higher animals has to be performed.

## Storage of PDLSC

It has recently been shown that PDLSC can be recovered from periodontal ligament tissues that have been cryopreserved for 3 or 6 months and still retain their stem cell characteristics and ability to regenerate PDL tissue when transplanted into immunocompromised mice. The cryopreserved PDLSC also showed that they had maintained the ability to differentiate into its three lineages, showed no difference in histology when compared to the fresh PDL and also expressed positive markers associated with PDLSC.

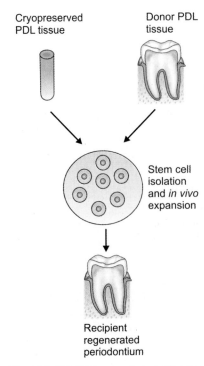

**Fig. 9.24:** PDLSC from periodontal ligament

A notable difference was that cryopreserved PDLSC when compared to fresh cultured PDLSC formed less single colonies when cultured. Further research in determining whether it was the time of storage that caused this depletion in colonies and if there is a maximum time limit allowed to store these stem cells is still needed. This evidence of PDLSC being able to be cryopreserved and still maintain their characteristics opens up the possibility of storing these stem cells for an extended period of time in case they are needed in a future transplant to a patient. As an added bonus, the ease in which cryopreservation of the PDL tissue has been performed can give future insight into creating a protocol that can be used for storing other tissues that contain stem cells.

### Future Studies

There still remains a lot that has to be learned about PDLSC. An experiment on the exact number of PDLSC that exists and the exact location of these stem cells within PDL tissues is still needed. The experiments that have been performed so far, have taken PDL tissue from extracted teeth, cultured this tissue to favor the expansion of PDLSC and then identified markers of PDLSC within the culture to guarantee quality. However, a specific structure of the periodontal ligament at the cellular level has not been created. More information is still needed on what conditions and cytokines favor *in vivo* differentiation of PDLSC into the different types of tissues within the periodontium. Although there are some protein factors that are known to play a role in differentiation of PDLSC, the specific pathway is not understood yet.

Another study that still has to be performed is the discovery of specific markers for PDLSC. Currently, markers that are found within mesenchymal stem cells are used to distinguish PDLSC. These markers are also found at variable levels within the PDL tissue, further illustrating that the PDL tissue is heterogenic and composed of cells that are found at different points of the differentiation process. The heterogeneous nature of the PDL tissue also brings up another important topic that has to be looked into further, which is the difference in the properties of the stem cells in perspective donors and recipients. This difference in properties could be a possible source of an immune response in a case where the PDLSC is transplanted to two people who have a significant difference amongst the properties of the stem cell.

As mentioned earlier, experiments have been done to cryopreserve the PDL while still keeping the tissue viable for later use of the PDLSCs. Another piece of information that is still needed is the maximum length of cryopreservation storage that is possible for PDL tissue and still capable of supporting PDLSC that can differentiate into their lineages. Due to the fact that PDL tissue is so easy to obtain from a variety of donors, these cells can be used to optimize cryopreservation techniques and the techniques may later be applied to other types of stem cells. This makes the PDL very important not just for the study of PDLSCs but also for other types of stem cells. PDLSC are mesenchymal stem cells so studies that are done with them may also apply to other mesenchymal stem cells which are more difficult to obtain due to more invasive procedures. People have their wisdom teeth removed everyday, which opens up an untapped source of stem cells from a variety of donors, without having to face the ethical issues involved with the procurement of many other types of stem cells.

### Conclusion

Periodontal disease is a worldwide problem that affects people of all classes. It is caused by a bacterial infection of the periodontium and results in a degeneration of tissue. Current methods used to repair any damage due to periodontal disease have poor efficacy, can be harmful, painful and expensive. The future therapeutic methods may involve tissue engineering using stem cells found in the periodontal ligament. The reason that the PDLSCs hold such great importance is that most of the cells are able to differentiated into a mixture of periodontal ligament—including the specific fiber bundles that attach tooth to bone and the mineralized tissue called cementum that covers the roots of our teeth. These cells are also beneficial in a clinical point of view because they are so easily accessible. In theory, people could one day preserve these stem cells and bank them from their own wisdom teeth that they have had extracted. These can then be used later in life to treat advanced periodontal disease. The idea of preserving one's own cells for later use is the ideal for the future of tissue engineering via stem cells.

## CLINICAL APPLICATION OF STEM CELLS IN OROFACIAL COMPLEX

Transplanted skeletal or dental stem cells may one day be used to repair craniofacial bone or even repair or regenerate teeth. While most often due to post-cancer ablative surgery, craniofacial osseous deficiencies can also arise from infection, trauma, congenital malformations, and progressive deforming skeletal diseases. Techniques used to repair craniofacial skeletal defects parallel the accepted surgical therapies for bone loss elsewhere in the skeleton and include the use of autogenous bone and alloplastic materials. However, despite the usefulness of these reparative strategies, each method has inherent limitations that restrict their universal application **(Fig. 9.25)**.

Transplantation of a bone marrow stromal cell population that contains skeletal stem cells may provide a promising alternative approach for reconstruction of craniofacial defects by circumventing many of the limitations of auto- and allografting methods. To date, most studies have shown the effectiveness of stem cell regenerative therapy in experimental animal models. In this strategy, stem cells are expanded in the laboratory, loaded onto an appropriate carrier, and locally transplanted to the site of a bony defect. Successful regeneration of bony defects that would not otherwise heal by cells in the local microenvironment has been shown in both calvarial and long bones models. Because of these successful findings in animal models, several centers are embarking on clinical trials to regenerate bone in humans.

## CHALLENGES IN CRANIOFACIAL TISSUE ENGINEERING

The relationship between bone marrow MSCs and the newly identified stem cells from various craniofacial tissues needs to be defined. In many ways, the newly characterized craniofacial stem cells resemble bone marrow MSCs, especially in terms of their differentiation capacities.

- Whether craniofacial-derived MSCs more effectively regenerate craniofacial structures than do appendicular MSCs needs to be explored.
- Whether craniofacial-derived MSCs are capable of healing noncraniofacial defects more effectively than appendicular MSCs also warrants investigation.
- How mechanical stress modulates craniofacial morphogenesis and regeneration needs to be further explored.
- The extent to which tissue engineering should mimic or recapitulate the corresponding developmental events needs to be determined.

## TISSUE ENGINEERING OF TEETH USING ADULT STEM CELLS

In order to tissue engineering of a tooth, it is necessary to understand the processes that lead to the induction and regulation of tooth development. Odontogenesis, in common with the development of most other organs, is a process that occurs within developing embryos via sequential and reciprocal interactions between mesenchymal and epithelial cells. Prior to odontogenesis, migratory cranial neural crest cells have a central role in the formation of the facial primordia, including the branchial arches. Neural crest cell migration commences early during development of the

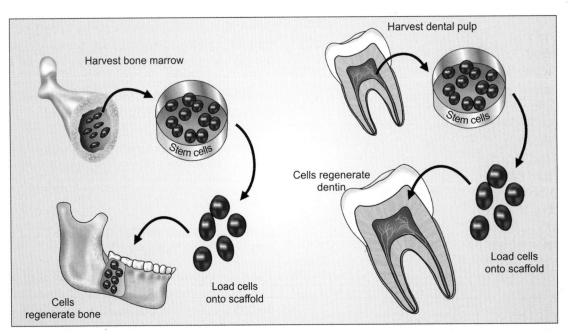

**Fig. 9.25:** Adult stem cells can be harvested from the bone marrow or dental tissues such as the dental pulp and expanded in the laboratory. When loaded onto appropriate scaffolds and transplanted back into a efficient site, stem cells have the potential to regenerate bone and tooth structures

embryo, at the head-fold stage. The jaw primordia are formed by neural crest cells emigrating from rhombomere-1 and the posterior region of the mesencephalon.

In the mouse, odontogenesis is induced around E10.0 when signals, largely in the form of protein ligands, are sent from the oral epithelium of the developing oral cavity to the underlying (ecto) mesenchyme. Fgf8, expressed in the oral epithelium, induces the expression of homeobox genes such as Barx1, Dlx1/2, Lhx6, Lhx7 and Pax9 in the ectomesenchyme. Bmp4, also expressed in the oral epithelium, induces the expression of the homeobox gene Msx1 in the ectomesenchyme while repressing the expression of Barx1 and Pax9. The expression domains of the homeobox genes coordinate the temporospatial development of the teeth. The co-expression of Lhx7, Msx1 and Pax9 is unique to odontogenic ectomesenchyme and hence their expression can be used as molecular markers of the induction of early tooth development.

The principles of early odontogenesis are being used to devise methods to generate teeth that can be used for replacement in humans. Our approach is to replace embryonic cells that make teeth in the embryo with cultured cells that can be isolated from a patient. Recombinant explants are produced from pellets of cells of nondental origin replacing the ectomesenchymal cells of the mandibular primordium. Cells used to date include neural stem cells taken from E14.0 spinal cords, embryonic stem cells and adult bone marrow cells. Embryonic Mandibular epithelium from GFP mice at stage E10.0 are placed on top of aggregates of these stem cells (Fig. 1) and cultured *in vitro* for 1 to 3 days. The expression of the early mesenchymal odontogenic marker genes, Lhx7, Msx1 and Pax9 in the Mesenchyme of normally developing mandibles, was detected in the cell aggregates adjacent to the epithelium. Negative controls, where cell pellets consisted of C3H10T1/2 and NIH3T3 cells which have no stem cell properties, did not show the induction of mesenchymal odontogenic molecular markers. Explants were also placed under renal capsules to determine if the early signs of odontogenesis, determined by observation of molecular markers, could be encouraged to develop further and produce a tooth. The environment within the renal capsule supplies the cells with the correct physiological conditions, including an adequate blood supply for longer term development.

Explants were grown in kidney capsules for 10-14 days after which they were removed and observed both histologically and with molecular markers. Recombination

between epithelium with neural stem cells, ES cells and bone marrow cells resulted in the production of soft tissues and bone. In several recombinant explants involving ES cells and neural stem cells the presence of Dspp, which is highly expressed in odontoblasts, was detected using radioactive *in situ* hybridisation. This indicates that although there were no recognisable teeth formed, there was tooth tissue present. Teeth were formed in three of the recombinant explants involving bone marrow cells cultured under renal capsules **(Figs 9.26A to D)**. This shows that the progenitor cells from the bone marrow were able to participate in odontogenesis as dental mesenchyme at E11.5 during normal odontogenesis. Negative controls for these renal capsule experiments consisted of C3H10T1/2 cells recombined with epithelium, NIH3T3 cell pellets recombined with epithelium, oral epithelium alone and stem cell pellets without epithelium. None of these produced teeth or tooth tissues. Implantation of tooth rudiments into the diastema.

If tooth germs or teeth are grown or cultured prior to implantation, it will be crucial to establish a method for implanting these into the mouth. To determine whether it would be possible to implant tooth germs successfully into oral mucosa in such a way that they continue to develop, E14.5 molar tooth rudiments were dissected and surgically implanted into the soft tissue of the diastema region of the maxilla of adult mice. The rudiments were allowed to grow for 26 days before removal for histological analysis. The implanted tooth germs were found to have developed into teeth of normal size connected to the bone by a differentiating connective tissue.

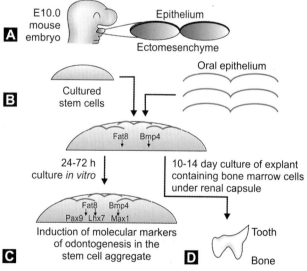

**Figs 9.26A to D:** Recombinant explants

The application of tissue engineering approaches in regenerative medicine and dentistry is an area of increasing interest and activity. Teeth have two major advantages over most other organs in that they are non-essential for life and easily accessible. Thus, teeth (and possibly also hair) are likely to be among the first organs that may provide a "proof of principle" for tissue engineered replacement organs. Crucial to being able to create replacement teeth is an understanding of their developmental biology and easily accessible sources of cells **(Fig. 9.27)**.

Control and prediction of tooth shape in the tissue engineered *in vitro* primordium will be a crucial step and one where developmental knowledge will be essential. Replacement of missing teeth with "natural" tissue engineered teeth in humans is some way off and indeed may prove too difficult, irreproducible or expensive. However, there is a real possibility that this will be achievable and, although there are no guarantees, what we learn along the way will be invaluable in our understanding of tooth development and stem cell biology.

## Stem Cells for Tooth Engineering

### Introduction

Teeth are highly mineralized organs resulting from sequential and reciprocal interactions between the oral epithelium and the underlying cranial neural crest-derived mesenchyme.

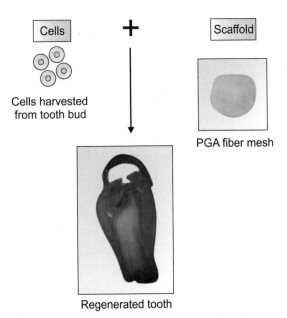

**Fig. 9.27:** Regenerated tooth by tissue engineering

Tissue recombination experiments point out that the oral epithelium contains the inductive capability for odontogenesis. This potential allows conditioning of the underlying mesenchyme, which in turn regulates the differentiation of epithelial cells. The importance of cranial neural crest-derived cells in odontogenesis has been shown in experiments where transplantation of mouse neural crest cells into chick embryos allowed growth of tooth germs. Numerous growth factors have been shown to be involved in different stages of the embryonic tooth development (i.e. initiation, morphogenesis, cytodifferentiation).

Members of the transforming growth factor beta (TGF-ß) superfamily such as bone morphogenic protein 2 (BMP-2) and BMP- 4 are key signalling molecules in regulating epithelial- mesenchymal interactions during odontogenesis. Molecules of the fibroblast growth factor (FGF) family such as FGF-3, FGF-4, FGF-8 and FGF-10 are involved in cell proliferation and regulate expression of specific target genes in teeth. Wnt proteins such as Wnt-3, Wnt-7b, Wnt-10a and Wnt-10b have essential roles as regulators of cell proliferation, migration and differentiation during tooth initiation and morphogenesis. Other diffusible factors such as sonic hedgehog (shh) also contribute to both initiation and subsequent dental morphogenesis. Two major cell types are involved in dental hard tissue formation: the mesenchyme-originated odontoblasts that are responsible for the production of dentin and the epithelium-derived ameloblasts that form the enamel. Odontoblasts are columnar postmitotic cells that form a layer in contact with the dentin. Odontoblastic processes are formed at their distal part, penetrate the dentin and participate in the secretion of dentin matrix and minerals. The matrix is composed of collagen (90%) and non-collagenous proteins such as Dentin Sialophosphoprotein (DSPP) and Dentin Matrix Protein 1 (DMP-1). The deposition of apatite minerals on this matrix gives rise to the mature calcified dentin. Enamel is secreted by ameloblasts along the dentino-enamel junction.

Enamel is mainly composed of hydrophobic proteins such as amelogenin, ameloblastin, enamelin, amelotin, tuftelin and ODAM (odontogenic ameloblast associated proteins). Shortly after enamel deposition, the formation of the root starts as a consequence of cell proliferation in the inner and outer dental epithelia at the cervical loop area. Cells from the dental follicle give rise to cementoblasts (forming the cementum that covers the dentin of the root), fibroblasts (generating the periodontal ligament) and osteoblasts (elaborating the alveolar bone). Cementum, periodontal ligament and alveolar bone are the periodontal tissues that support teeth into the oral cavity. Tooth loss or absence is a common and frequent situation that can result from numerous pathologies such as periodontal and carious diseases, fractures, injuries or even genetic alterations. In most cases this loss is not critical, but for aesthetical, psychological and medical reasons (e.g. genetic aberrations) replacement of the missing teeth is important.

Recent efforts made in the field of biomaterials have led to the development of dental implants composed of biocompatible materials such as titanium that can be inserted in the maxillary and/or mandibular bone to replace the missing teeth. However, implants are still not completely satisfactory and their successful use greatly depends on their osteointegration. The quantity and quality of the bone, as well as its interaction with the surface of the implant are some crucial parameters that can influence the achievement of the operation. Although innovative materials and techniques (e.g. surface treatment) have been used for the improvement of implant osteointegration, the metal/bone interface does not ensure complete integration of the implant, thus reducing its performance and long-term stability. Furthermore, dental implant technology is dependent on bone volume, as devices (i.e. peg) can be implanted only in patients possessing a sufficient amount of bone. Quite often there is a need for alveolar bone volume increase before any implant fixing. To overcome these difficulties, new ideas and approaches have emerged recently from the quickly developing fields of stem cell technology and tissue engineering **(Fig. 9.28)**.

## Stem Cells in Regenerative Medicine

A stem cell is defined as a cell that can continuously produce unaltered daughters and, furthermore, has the ability to generate cells with different and more restricted properties. Stem cells can divide either symmetrically (allowing the increase of stem cell number) or asymmetrically. Asymmetric divisions keep the number of stem cells unaltered and are responsible for the generation of cells with different properties. These cells can either multiply (progenitors or transit amplifying cells) or be committed to terminal differentiation. Progenitors and transit amplifying cells have a limited lifespan and therefore can only reconstitute a tissue for a short period of time when transplanted. In contrast, stem cells are self-renewing and thus can generate any tissue for a lifetime. This is a key property for a successful therapy. The capacity to expand stem cells in culture is an indispensable step for regenerative medicine, and a considerable effort has been

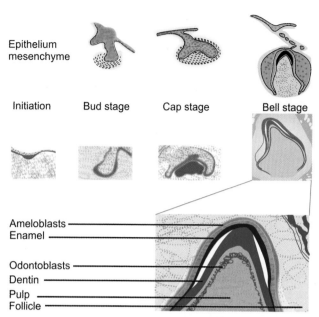

**Fig. 9.28:** Schematic illustration and histological sections showing the different stages of tooth development in humans. The sections were stained with hematoxylin. Orange color indicates epithelial tissues and epithelial derivatives (ameloblasts and enamel) while blue color shows mesenchymal tissues and mesenchyme derivatives (odontoblasts, dentin, dental pulp and follicle)

made to evaluate the consequences of the cultivation on stem cell behavior.

Stem cells cannot be identified with certainty in any tissue: scientists rely on indirect properties such as the expression of a repertoire of surface proteins, slow cell cycle, clonogenicity, or an undifferentiated state. However, none of these criteria are specific. The evaluation of self-renewal is the ultimate way to show "stemness", which relies on the isolation and transplantation of a putative stem cell (clonal analysis) followed by its serial transplantation and long-term reconstitution of a tissue. During recent years, stem cells have been used extensively in many medical disciplines for the repair and/ or regeneration of defective tissues and organs (e.g. bone, ligament, heart). New therapeutic approaches are largely inspired and based on our knowledge of embryonic development.

Schematic illustration and histological sections showing the different stages of tooth development in humans. The sections were stained with hematoxylin. Orange color indicates epithelial tissues and epithelial derivatives (ameloblasts and enamel) while blue color shows mesenchymal tissues and mesenchyme derivatives (odontoblasts, dentin, dental pulp and follicle).

The aim of regenerative medicine is to stepwise re-create *in vitro* all the mechanisms and processes that nature uses during initiation and morphogenesis of a given organ. In this context, stem cell research offers an amazing and seductive potential for body homeostasis, repair, regeneration and pathology. The possibility of manipulating stem cells *in situ* using specific signalling molecules or by expanding them *ex vivo* is an exciting outcome of basic research. Hence, regenerative medicine has become a fashionable field and the isolation and manipulation of embryonic and adult (or postnatal) stem cells for the creation of new functional organs that will replace the missing or defective organs constitutes an enormous challenge. Embryonic and adult stem cells have been under intense investigation that focuses on the *in vitro* development of new organs such as hair, skin and bone. Adult stem cells (ASCs), which possess a restricted potential of differentiation, can easily be isolated from a patient and after *in vitro* amplification and/or differentiation could be re-injected to the same patient thus avoiding immune rejection, as is the case for allografts or xenografts. Since numerous problems remain, the ideal protocol for human pathologies is far away from being used. However, the knowledge in stem cell technology is increasing quickly in all medical disciplines and dictates the need for new strategic approaches in all fields, including reparative dentistry. Stem cell therapy constitutes a common challenge for dentists as well as biologists.

### Dental Stem Niches and Other Stem Cell Sources for the Development of Teeth in vitro or ex vivo

As tooth formation results from epithelial-mesenchymal interactions, two different populations of stem cells have to be considered: epithelial stem cells (EpSCs), which will give rise to ameloblasts, and mesenchymal stem cells (MSCs) that will form the odontoblasts, cementoblasts, osteoblasts and fibroblasts of the periodontal ligament. Thus, tooth engineering using stem cells is based on their isolation, association and culture as recombinants *in vitro* or *ex vivo* conditions to assess firstly tooth morphogenesis and secondly cell differentiation into tooth specific cells that will form dentin, enamel, cementum and alveolar bone. Various approaches could be used according to the origin of stem cells.

Many recent studies have focused on the localization of sites of adult tissues/organs where specific ASC populations reside. ASC are quiescent, slow-cycling, undifferentiated cells, which are surrounded by neighboring cells and extracellular matrix. This microenvironment is specific for each stem cell compartment but is likely to be influenced by common factors such as vasculature or loading pressure. The specialized microenvironment, housing ASC and transient-amplifying cells (TACs), forms a "niche". Understanding these microenvironments and their regulation is the key for the successful reproduction of such niches and for the *ex vivo* engineering of an organ with ensured functional homeostasis. In teeth, two different stem cell niches have been suggested: the cervical loop of rodent incisor for EpSC and a perivascular niche in adult dental pulp for MSC. In rodent incisors the proliferation of EpSC, which is located at the cervical loop area, is governed by signals from the surrounding mesenchyme. FGF signalling (mainly FGF-3 and FGF-10) is of particular importance since it is linked to the Notch pathway. Molecules such as BMPs, Activin and Follistatin are also expressed inside the stem cell niche and are known to regulate it's maintenance and functionality through a complex integrative network. In the dental pulp, MSCs are thought to reside in a perivascular niche, but little is known on the exact location and molecular regulation of this niche. The Eph receptor tyrosine kinase family of guidance molecules appears to be involved in the maintenance of the human dental pulp perivascular niche. Eph-B and its ligand Ephrin-B were shown to inhibit MSC migration and attachment via the MAPK pathway through unidirectional and bidirectional signalling respectively. In addition to the dental pulp MSC, other MSC populations have been isolated from human dental tissues such as the periodontal ligament and the dental follicle, but nothing is known about the existence of a niche in these tissues.

### Mesenchymal Stem Cells

MSC can be isolated from different sources. First described in bone marrow, MSC have been extensively characterized *in vitro* by the expression of markers such as STRO-1, CD146 or CD44. STRO-1 is a cell surface antigen used to identify osteogenic precursors in bone marrow, CD146 a pericyte marker, and CD44 a mesenchymal stem cell marker. MSC possess a high self-renewal capacity and the potential to differentiate into mesodermal lineages thus forming cartilage, bone, adipose tissue, skeletal muscle and the stroma of connective tissues. The potential of dental MSC for tooth regeneration and repair has been extensively studied in the last years. Below, we discuss mesenchymal progenitors that have been assessed for tooth engineering purposes, such as progenitors derived from teeth and bone marrow.

## Stem Cells from Human Exfoliated Deciduous Teeth (SHED)

The isolation of postnatal stem cells from an easily accessible source is indispensable for tissue engineering and clinical applications. Recent findings demonstrated the isolation of mesenchymal progenitors from the pulp of human deciduous incisors. These cells were named SHED (stem cells from human exfoliated deciduous teeth) and exhibited a high plasticity since they could differentiate into neurons, adipocytes, osteoblasts and odontoblasts. *In vivo* SHED cells can induce bone or dentin formation but, in contrast to dental pulp, DPSC failed to produce a dentin-pulp complex.

## Adult Dental Pulp Stem Cells (DPSCs)

After a dental injury, dental pulp is involved in a process called reparative dentinogenesis, where cells elaborate and deposit a new dentin matrix for the repair of the injured site. It has been shown that adult dental pulp contains precursors capable of forming odontoblasts under appropriate signals. Among these signals are the calcium hydroxide or calcium phosphate materials, which constitute pulp-capping materials used by dentists for common dental treatments. Dental pulp progenitors have not been clearly identified but some data suggest that pericytes, which are able to differentiate into osteoblasts, could also differentiate into odontoblasts. Tooth repair is a lifetime process thus suggesting that MSC might exist in adult dental pulp. The *in vivo* therapeutic targeting of these adult stem cells remains to be explored.

## Stem Cells from the Apical Part of the Papilla (SCAP)

Stem cells from the apical part of the human dental papilla (SCAP) have been isolated and their potential to differentiate into odontoblasts was compared to that of the periodontal ligament stem cells (PDLSCs). SCAP exhibit a higher proliferative rate and appears more effective than PDLSC for tooth formation. Importantly, SCAP are easily accessible since they can be isolated from human third molars. Stem cells from the dental follicle (DFSC). DFSC have been isolated from follicle of human third molars and express the stem cell markers Notch1, STRO-1 and nestin. These cells can be maintained in culture for at least 15 passages. STRO-1 positive DFSC can differentiate into cementoblasts *in vitro* and are able to form cementum *in vivo*. Immortalized dental follicle cells are able to recreate a new periodontal ligament (PDL) after *in vivo* implantation.

## Periodontal Ligament Stem Cells (PDLSCs)

The PDL is a specialized tissue located between the cementum and the alveolar bone and has as a role the maintenance and support of the teeth. Its continuous regeneration is thought to involve mesenchymal progenitors arising from the dental follicle. PDL contains STRO-1 positive cells that maintain certain plasticity since they can adopt adipogenic, osteogenic and chondrogenic phenotypes *in vitro*. It is thus obvious that PDL itself contains progenitors, which can be activated to self-renew and regenerate other tissues such as cementum and alveolar bone.

## Bone Marrow Derived Mesenchymal Stem Cells (BMSCs)

BMSC have been tested for their ability to recreate periodontal tissue. These cells are able to form *in vivo* cementum, PDL and alveolar bone after implantation into defective periodontal tissues. Thus, bone marrow provides an alternative source of MSC for the treatment of periodontal diseases. BMSC share numerous characteristics with DPSC and are both able to form bone-like or tooth-like structures. However, BMSC display a lower odontogenic potential than DPSC, indicating that MSC from different embryonic origins are not equivalent. Indeed, DPSC derive from neural crest cells, whereas BMSC originate from the mesoderm. Furthermore, the comparison of the osteogenic and adipogenic potential of MSC from different origins shows that, even if cells carry common genetic markers, they are not equivalent and are already committed toward a specific differentiation pathway. Commitment could arise from conditioning of stem cells by their specific micro-environment or stem cell niche. MSC can also be obtained from several other sources such as synovial and periosteum. As these cell populations display distinctive biological properties depending upon their tissue of origin, it remains to be explored which source might be used for an optimal tooth development for clinical application.

## In Search of Epithelium Originated Dental Stem Cells

Although significant progress has been made with MSC, there is no information available for dental EpSC in humans. The major problem is that dental epithelial cells such as ameloblasts and ameloblasts precursors are eliminated soon after tooth eruption. Therefore, epithelial cells that could be stimulated *in vivo* to form enamel are not present in human adult teeth. Stem cell technology appears to be the only possibility to recreate an enamel surface.

### Epithelial Stem Cells from Developing Molars

Several studies describe the use of EpSC isolated from newborn or juvenile animals, usually from third molar teeth. In these studies, epithelia were removed and cells dissociated enzymatically. Precursors were then amplified and associated with MSC (originated from the same tooth) *in vitro* in contact with biomaterials such as collagen sponges or synthetic polymers. These approaches are promising for tooth formation and/or regeneration. However, the clinical application is difficult, if not unrealistic, since it would require the donation of a tooth germ from children. The use of autologous stem cells is desirable but raises the question of a good and reliable source.

### Epithelial Stem Cells from the Labial Cervical Loop of Rodent Incisor

The rodent incisor is a unique model for studying dental EpSC since, in contrast to human incisors or other vertebrates, this tooth grows throughout life. An EpSC niche, which is located in the apical part of the rodent incisor epithelium (cervical loop area), is responsible for a continuous enamel matrix production. In this highly proliferative area, undifferentiated epithelial cells migrate toward the anterior part of the incisor and give rise to ameloblasts. Although these findings are important for understanding the mechanisms of stem cell homing, renewal and differentiation, this source of dental EpSC cannot be used for treatment in humans since it would require the introduction of rodent cells in the human mouth.

Dental EpSC can be isolated from postnatal teeth but exhibit complex problems that strongly limit their clinical application in humans. Other sources are thus required. Ideally these sources should be easily accessible, available from adult individuals and the derived cells must have potential for enamel matrix production. The use of non-dental EpSC will only be possible with the transfer of genes, creating an odontogenic potential to non-dental epithelia prior to any association with mesenchymal cells. This is certainly one of the most exciting goals of the next decade in tooth engineering **(Fig. 9.29)**.

### Association of Epithelial and Mesenchymal Stem Cells

Since teeth are formed from two different tissues, building a tooth logically requires the association/cooperation of odontogenic mesenchymal and epithelial cells. The recombination of dissociated dental epithelial and mesenchymal tissues leads to tooth formation both *in vitro* and *in vivo*. Numerous attempts have been made in order to form teeth *in vivo* with very promising results. Single cell suspensions

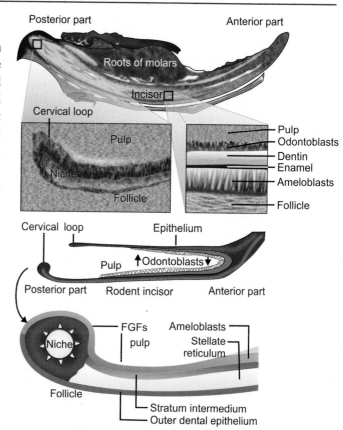

**Fig. 9.29:** Histological sections and schematic representation of a mandibular rodent incisor. The sections were stained with hematoxylin/ eosin. Epithelial stem cells located in the cervical loop area (posterior part of the incisor) migrate towards the anterior part of the incisor and give rise to four epithelial cell layers: ameloblasts, stratum intermedium, stellate reticulum and outer dental epithelium

obtained from rat, pig or mice tooth germs have been seeded onto the surface of selected biomaterials (e.g. collagen-coated polyglycolic acid, calcium phosphate material, collagen sponges) and successfully reimplanted into the omentum of immunocompromised animals. All these reports describe the presence of both dentin and enamel. This indicates that the recombined cells could reorganize themselves and form individual layers and, furthermore, that they can differentiate properly into *odontoblasts* and *ameloblasts*.

In most of these studies, the cells were directly seeded onto biomaterials without any additional *in vitro* procedure. In studies including *in vitro* steps before the *in vivo* transplantation, the results could be influenced by several critical parameters such as the presence or absence of serum, the type of serum, the composition of culture media, the cell density and the ratio between epithelial and mesenchymal cells. For these reasons, a definitive and universal protocol for tooth formation does not exist so far. Making entire teeth with enamel and dentin structures *in vivo* is a reality and not a utopia. However, these bioengineered teeth have been produced in ectopic sites and are still missing some essential elements such as the complete root and periodontal tissues that allow correct anchoring into the alveolar bone. Recently, a new approach has been proposed for growing teeth in the mouse mandible. In this study, epithelial and mesenchymal cells were sequentially seeded into a collagen gel drop and then implanted into the tooth cavity of adult mice. With this technique the presence of all dental structures such as odontoblasts, ameloblasts, dental pulp,blood vessels, crown, periodontal ligament, root and alveolar bone could be observed. Thus, the implantation of these tooth germs in the mandible allowed their development, maturation and eruption (**Fig. 9.30**) indicating that stem cells could be used in the future for the replacement of missing teeth in humans.

Despite the outstanding advances in tooth bioengineering, such a technology cannot be applied to human

restorative dentistry for one simple reason: the epithelial and mesenchymal cells used for tooth reconstruction are of dental origin and have been given by a donor. The challenge that remains is to find out new and easily accessible sources of both epithelial and mesenchymal stem cells that can be reprogrammed for an odontogenic potential and then associated to form a fully functional tooth. One alternative could be the use of genetically modified cells expressing specific genes (e.g. transgenes, siRNA) or with a specifically deleted gene (e.g. knock-in, knock-out). Ideally, this approach should provide a nonlimited source of cells and introduce new genetic information to reprogram a nondental cell to acquire odontogenic properties. For example, p53-deficient mice were used to establish dental epithelial clonal cell lines subsequently associated with mesenchymal cells to bioengineer teeth *in vivo*. These cell lines demonstrated heterogeneous outcomes in terms of regeneration depending on their differentiation state. Although this technique provides

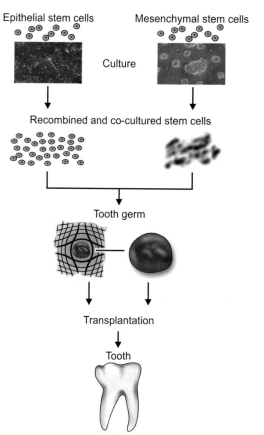

**Fig. 9.30:** Use of stem cells for tooth formation *in vitro* and *ex vivo*. A tooth germ can be created *in vitro* after co-culture of isolated epithelial and mesenchymal stem cells. This germ could be implanted into the alveolar bone and finally develop into a fully functional tooth.

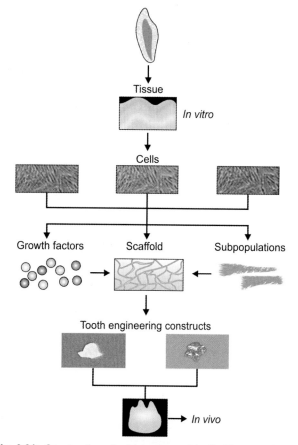

**Fig. 9.31:** Construction of a bioengineered tooth. The association of tooth-derived stem cells with defined scaffolds in the presence of growth factors allows the creation of tooth specific constructs such as crown and root of missing parts of an injured tooth. These biological constructs could be used in dental clinics as substitutes for metal implants, crowns and restorative dental materials.

us with an unlimited source of epithelial cells and shows the potential of genetically modified cells that can be used for tooth engineering, many questions have to be resolved. Which gene should be used to trigger an odontogenic program? Is only one gene enough to reprogram a cell toward a tooth specific cell?

### Conclusion

Taken together these recent findings clearly indicate that the control of morphogenesis and cytodifferentiation is a challenge that necessitates a thorough understanding of the cellular and molecular events involved in development, repair and regeneration of teeth. The identification of several types of epithelial and mesenchymal stem cells in the tooth and the knowledge of molecules involved in stem cell fate is a significant achievement. *In vitro* and *in vivo* experiments using these cells have provided promising results illustrated by the generation of a complete tooth with all dental structures including cells and extracellular matrix deposition. However, many problems remain to be addressed before considering the clinical use of these technologies. The use of animal cells for human diseases is restricted by immune rejection risks.

Additionally, isolating autologous stem cells requires a source of easily accessible cells without the need for a surgery. It may be possible to replace dental mesenchymal stem cells with stem cells of another origin. At present, it does not appear that this is the case for epithelial stem cells. A reliable source of EpSC for that purpose remains to be determined. Alternative solutions such as the use of artificial crowns are considered. The engineering of tri-dimensional matrices (either polylactic acid polymers or collagen sponges) which a composition more or less similar to that of the organs to reconstruct, and the addition of growth factors such as FGF, BMP or PDGF might facilitate the transplantation and the differentiation of stem cells **(Fig. 9.31)**. However, the engineering of tooth substitutes is hard to scale up, costly, time-consuming and incompatible with the treatment of extensive tooth loss. Scientific knowledge is not enough and the main challenge in stem cell therapy is to find a compromise between the benefits to the patients, regulatory agencies, increased stem cell requirements, costs, coverage by health insurance and the role of pharmaceutical companies.

### Research Promise (Fig. 9.32)

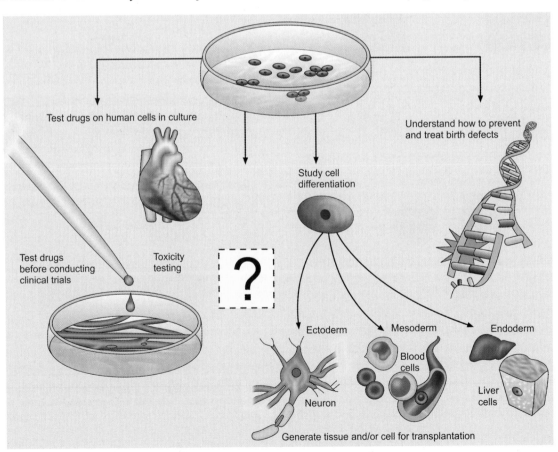

**Fig. 9.32:** The promise of stem cell research

# *Conclusion*

Stem cells are the primal cells found in all multicellular organisms. They are unspecialized cells that develop into the specialized cells that make up the different types of tissue in the human body. They are vital to the development, growth, maintenance, and repair of our brains, bones, muscles, nerves, blood, skin, and other organs. They retain the ability to renew them through mitotic cell division and can differentiate into a diverse range of specialized cell types. Stem cells are not far fetched science fiction, but one day it will become a part of every clinician practice. The immediate challenges for the researchers is not only to be better prepared to address the questions that their patients have concerning stem cell–based therapy, but also to familiarize themselves with the spectrum of tools they may have in the near future to restore form and function effectively.

As stem cells can be grown and transformed into specialized cells, with characteristics consistent with cells, of various tissues such as muscles or nerves through cell culture, their use in medical therapies has been proposed. In particular, embryonic cell lines, autologous embryonic stem cells generated through therapeutic cloning, and highly plastic adult stem cells from the umbilical cord blood or bone marrow are touted as promising candidates. In the laboratory, researchers are learning the ways to coax stem cells to differentiate into specialized kinds of cells, and to create the conditions under which stem cells will replicate themselves for extended periods of time. If these unique properties can be understood and harnessed, stem cells hold great potential as tools for medical research and as therapeutic agents.

Scientists are using stem cells to study basic processes of embryological development, including the processes that lead to genetic disease and abnormalities. They also are conducting research to see if stem cells might be used directly for therapeutic purposes. Given appropriate nutrients, stem cells can replicate in the laboratory without differentiating, and thus create stem cell lines. Such cell lines are valuable because they allow researchers to work with quantities of genetically identical material at different times and places.

Stem cell research and its applications hold scientific and medical promise. Like other powerful technologies, they pose challenges and risks as well. If we are to realize the benefits, meet the challenges, and avoid the risks, stem cell research must be conducted under effective, accountable systems of social oversight and control, at both national and international levels. The stem cell dogmas of yesterday are not withstanding the research findings of today, and many investigators are discovering that what once was is no longer relevant today.

In closing, the potential uses for stem cells seem endless. The ability to isolate and in some cases, culture adult stem cells lead to future hope in genetically correcting abnormal stem cells to treat various human genetic disorders, and to employ hematopoietic stem cell therapy to treat not only autoimmune diseases, but also a variety of different genetic disorders extending beyond those of the hematopoietic system. The generation of perfect "Dollys" for agricultural livestock represents another promising avenue of scientific research.

Even when this technology is taken just one small step further, the world still shudders at the potential moral and

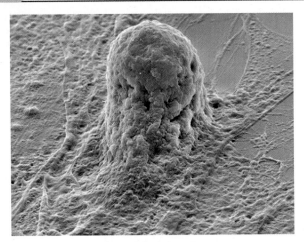

**Fig. 10.1:** Stem cells

ethical dangers of opening the Pandora's box of human reproductive cloning. The technology requirement of reproductive cloning is presently too low to be feasible for regenerating a lost child or loved one. Yet stem cell biology is advancing at an incredibly rapid pace, and with the powerful potential for this technology in the treatment and cure of various hitherto life-threatening disorders, the feasibility will soon be at our doorstep. It is thus imperative as we begin the next millenium, that our scientists sit at the round table with the rest of humanity and together face these very difficult moral and ethical concerns that touch the essence of life itself, the stem cell **(Fig. 10.1)**.

# *Index*